D1612311

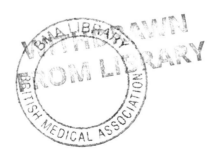

The Language of Mental Health

Series Editors
Michelle O'Reilly
The Greenwood Institute
University of Leicester
Leicester, UK

Jessica Nina Lester
School of Education
Indiana University
Bloomington, IN, USA

This series brings together rich theoretical and empirical discussion at the intersection of mental health and discourse/conversation analysis. Situated broadly within a social constructionist perspective, the books included within this series will offer theoretical and empirical examples highlighting the discursive practices that surround mental health and make 'real' mental health constructs. Drawing upon a variety of discourse and conversation analysis perspectives, as well as data sources, the books will allow scholars and practitioners alike to better understand the role of language in the making of mental health. Editorial board We are very grateful to our expert editorial board who continue to provide support for the book series. We are especially appreciative of the feedback that they have provided on earlier drafts of this book. Their supportive comments and ideas to improve the book have been very helpful in our development of the text. They continue to provide support as we continue to edit the book series 'the language of mental health'. We acknowledge them here in alphabetical order by surname. Tim Auburn, Plymouth University, UK; Galina Bolden, Rutgers University, USA; Susan Danby, Queensland University of Technology, Australia; Debra Friedman, Indiana University, USA; Ian Hutchby, University of Leicester, UK; Doug Maynard, University of Wisconsin, USA; Emily A. Nusbaum, University of San Francisco, USA.

More information about this series at
http://www.palgrave.com/gp/series/15193

Cordet Smart · Timothy Auburn
Editors

Interprofessional Care and Mental Health

A Discursive Exploration of Team Meeting Practices

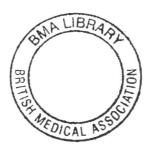

palgrave
macmillan

Editors
Cordet Smart
School of Psychology
University of Plymouth
Plymouth, UK

Timothy Auburn
School of Psychology
University of Plymouth
Plymouth, UK

The Language of Mental Health
ISBN 978-3-319-98227-4   ISBN 978-3-319-98228-1   (eBook)
https://doi.org/10.1007/978-3-319-98228-1

Library of Congress Control Number: 2018950735

Cover illustration: fotostorm/gettyimages

This Palgrave Macmillan imprint is published by the registered company Springer Nature Switzerland AG
The registered company address is: Gewerbestrasse 11, 6330 Cham, Switzerland

Acknowledgements

We would like to firstly thank our service user and carer group based at Plymouth University, for their comments on the research programme at intervals from its inception to its completion, and all of the service users and carers who have commented along the way, in particular Christianne Pollock, who we recognise as a carer who has had profound personal challenges to manage, and has still kindly and helpfully commented on our work and even found time to author some chapters.

Kind thanks also go to Jacqui Stedmon, Emma Newton and Nneamaka Ekebuisi for their hard work with reviewing chapters. Jacqui Stedmon is an Associate Lecturer and the Course Director of Plymouth University's Clinical Psychology Programme. She is a clinical psychologist specialising in children's mental health and bereavement and kindly reviewed Chapter 15 for us. Emma Newton and Nnemaka Ekebuisi are both currently third-year clinical psychology trainees and kindly took time out in their busy year to review chapters. Emma Newton reviewed several chapters including Chapters 5 and 7, and Nnemaka reviewed Chapter 3. We would also like to thank all of our participants for taking part in the research and engaging so fully in the process. In addition, we would like to thank our clinical commentators, including Dr. Jane Suzanne, a specialist clinical psychologist in Devon Partnership Trust, and Dr. Sarah Whittham, a specialist clinical psychologist in Cornwall Foundation NHS Trust. Both of these people have provided valuable insights and reflections around how the research worked.

Our research assistants have also worked hard, including Brajan Stovac, Holly Reed and Nancy Froomberg, all of whom have contributed to the organisation of the data and the administration of the project.

Contents

Notes on Contributors

Dr. Lindsay Aikman is working as a highly specialist clinical psychologist in an acute inpatient mental health unit in the UK. Before moving in to mental health in 2009, Lindsay spent almost ten years working internationally in management consultancy and specialised in team dynamics and organisational change. She now works in ways that blends these two fields, promoting the importance of interprofessional team working as a key factor in facilitating joined-up experiences of health and social care. Her commitment to this philosophy earned her an award from the Division of Clinical Psychology for co-founding an interdisciplinary learner-led initiative while completing her Doctorate in Clinical Psychology. An awareness of organisational systems and how they support best practice, innovation and change has continued to be of interest to Lindsay, noticing how differently MDT practices can be operationalised within services. Lindsay passionately believes that supporting clinicians to be the best versions of themselves is core to the sustainable delivery of compassionate care, and so nurturing compassionate working environments is central to her practice, and a research topic she presented on at the Compassionate Mind Foundation's 4th International Conference in 2015.

Timothy Auburn is an Associate Professor in the School of Psychology, University of Plymouth. He has had a long-standing interest in the uses of conversation analysis for understanding the way society's core institutions work and for promoting changes in these institutions at the level of interaction. As well as his current interest in multidisciplinary team meetings and their role in health care, his other research interests include problem-solving for offenders in the lower courts, and the barriers and outcomes of altruistic kidney donation.

Dominique Clancy is a third-year trainee clinical psychologist on the Doctorate in Clinical Psychology at the University of Plymouth. Her doctoral research is focused on exploring the experience of students attending Schwartz Rounds conducted in the University context. Dominique has a Master's in Forensic Psychology from the University of York and a Bachelor of Science with Honours in Psychology from the University of York. She was worked across child and adult mental health and learning disability services and has a keen interest in supporting the well-being of staff working in health care.

Emily Connolly is a trainee clinical psychologist at Plymouth University. She is interested in how reflective practice works within clinical practice, and is engaged in a number of interprofessional working initiatives. This includes the development of 'Bridges', where students from different professionals come together to enhance integrated learning and thinking.

Dr. Jennifer Dickenson is working as a clinical psychologist within an NHS older people's mental health service in the UK. She works within both community and inpatient MDTs who provide services both people with a diagnosis of dementia and people who are experiencing mental health difficulties. Jenny values MDT working and encourages psychological formulation within all aspects of her work.

Ben Durkin Peer Support Organisation, Exeter, UK.

Nancy Froomberg is a Research Assistant based at Plymouth University. Her interests lie in discourse analysis with a focus on conversational analysis as a methodology for examining the way in which language works and how we achieve social actions within this.

Dr. Sifiso Mhlanga is a clinical psychologist, currently working within an acute inpatient mental health service in the NHS. Her previous experience includes working within forensic and locked rehabilitation services in the NHS and in the private sector. Her current clinical and research interests include promoting a psychotherapeutic culture through facilitating reflective practice groups and providing colleagues with regular training informed by a variety of psychological approaches.

Nicole Parish is a clinical psychologist, currently working for the NHS within the Noah's Ark Children's Hospital for Wales. She is particularly interested in the benefits of interprofessional working and the use of psychological ideas to promote well-being within wide organisations such as hospitals and schools.

Dr. Katherine Peckitt is a Clinical Psychologist with a special interest in psychosis.

Christianne Pollock has a particular interest in learning disability and autism and has been involved in this project as an expert by experience. She has previously used Conversation Analysis to look at interactions of children with severe autism. She now runs a business providing Jeffersonian transcription for researchers and is currently training to be a speech and language therapist.

Holly Reed is a Research Assistant at Plymouth University. She received a British Psychological Society Undergraduate Award in 2017 to work on the *MDTsInAction* project and develop the work around topics related to advocacy.

Cordet Smart is a Lecturer in the School of Psychology, University of Plymouth. She is the Chief Investigator on the *MDTsInAction* research programme, which she developed combining her training as an Adult Nurse, Ph.D. in discourse and social influence in organisations, and extensive experience as a research tutor for 10 years on the Plymouth Clinical Psychology Training Programme, and gained from the Exeter Doctorate in Clinical Psychotherapy. She is particularly interested in examining interactions within clinical and group contexts (such as families and health care organisations) and exploring the multiple presentations of social influence from a discursive psychology perspective.

Ashley Tauchert Peer Support Organisation, Exeter, UK.

Brajan Sztorc is an undergraduate psychology student who has worked as a Research Assistant with Dr. Cordet Smart on this project.

Madeleine Tremblett is a Teaching and Research Associate at the University of Plymouth, completing her Ph.D. in between her teaching responsibilities for the School of Psychology. Her Ph.D. focuses on how multidisciplinary teams collaborate in Intellectual (Learning) Disability services. Drawing heavily on discursive methods to examine meetings held between professionals, Madeleine is interested in understanding how examining everyday interactions can help uncover practices used to provide effective care.

Dr. Claire Whiter is currently working as clinical psychologist within a multidisciplinary Community Mental Health Team. She has used mental health services herself and has worked across statutory and voluntary sectors within the fields of teaching, women's mental health and Early Intervention in Psychosis Services. She is working to promote involvement of service users and carers across all levels of the mental health service and the application of involvement within the research process. Within her clinical work, Claire is interested in psychological approaches to working with psychosis and finding an elaborated language for emotionality and distress that may be shared by service users, carers and staff. Her clinical and research interests lie in feminist approaches to mental health including consideration of social inequalities and qualitative methodologies.

Erica Willoughby is an Assistant Psychologist in a community adult learning disabilities team. Prior to this Erica completed a masters degree, under the supervision of Dr. Cordet Smart, with her thesis focusing on observing power in MDTs.

Abbreviations

ADHD	Attention Deficit Hyperactivity Disorder
ADI	Autism Diagnostic Inventory
ADOS	Autism Diagnostic Observation Schedule
ASD	Autism Spectrum Disorder
BPS	British Psychological Society
CA	Conversation Analysis
CDP	Critical Discursive Psychology
CMHN	Community Mental Health Nurse
CMHT	Community Mental Health Team
CPN	Community Psychiatric Nurse
DA	Discourse Analysis
DP	Discursive Psychology
DSM	Diagnostic and Statistical Manual
EI	Early Intervention in Psychosis
IAPT	Improving Access to Psychological Therapies
IDK	'I Don't Know' Utterances
ILD	Intellectual Learning Disability
IPE	Interprofessional Education
IPL	Interprofessional Learning
LD	Learning Disability
MD	Medical Doctor

MDT	Multidisciplinary Team
OCD	Obsessive Compulsive Disorder
OT	Occupational Therapist
PLD	Person living with dementia
PPI	Public and Patient Involvement
QAA	Quality Assurance Agency
SALT	Speech and Language Therapist
TCU	Turn Construction Unit
TRP	Transition Relevance Place

List of Tables

1

Introduction: Problems and Prospects for Multidisciplinary Team Meetings

Cordet Smart, Jennifer Dickenson, Timothy Auburn and Nancy Froomberg

Introduction

Imagine a world where we could all just sit together at a table and instantly produce the perfect solution for every service user that we are presented with. Well that is probably not going to happen. But the alternative is that we sit around a table and never agree to anything.

C. Smart (✉) · T. Auburn · N. Froomberg
School of Psychology, University of Plymouth, Plymouth, UK
e-mail: cordet.smart@plymouth.ac.uk

T. Auburn
e-mail: T.Auburn@plymouth.ac.uk

N. Froomberg
e-mail: nancy.froomberg@plymouth.ac.uk

J. Dickenson
Devon Partnership NHS Trust, Exeter, UK
e-mail: jenniferdickenson@nhs.net

© The Author(s) 2018
C. Smart and T. Auburn (eds.), *Interprofessional Care and Mental Health*,
The Language of Mental Health, https://doi.org/10.1007/978-3-319-98228-1_1

Over the last 100 years, there has been a proliferation of healthcare professionals, so that now we have occupational therapists, physiotherapists, nurses, clinical psychologists, psychiatrists, doctors of numerous forms, medical assistants, nursing assistants.... The list is endless. They each have different levels of training and speciality, but one professional requirement they all share is that they need to be able to work together. As this increased diversification has occurred, it is arguable that the importance of joined up, collaborative care has also increased. The service user, amid all of these would-be helpful people, has to be able to feel that these professionals are working in some form of coherent manner. This need for effective collaborative care in itself creates a dilemma for these different professionals—how to work together as a team whilst simultaneously maintaining their professional identity and autonomy.

This book specifically examines team working in various mental health contexts. Within mental healthcare settings, collaboration is essential to ensure that people feel confident in the care that they receive, and that anxiety levels or feelings of disengagement are not further exacerbated. Collaboration in mental health can require specific forms of communication that might not be as relevant in other areas of health care; for example, there are particular sensitivities concerning the ways to approach service users, or the how to support staff (Chong, Aslani, & Chen, 2013).

This book reports a research programme that examined in detail how interprofessional working is implemented in a range of mental health settings. We are particularly privileged to have been able to study interprofessional care at a unique point in time when service user involvement is increasingly valued, and so hope that this book will instigate a new generation of researchers to understand better all of its components. We would like people to understand the face-to-face aspects of interprofessional care, in particular how multidisciplinary team meetings are managed and organised by the people who actually take part in them. Our research programme conjoins advances in mental health care prioritising patient experience, a culture of service user and carer involvement and consultation in practice and research, with advances in the study of how language works as a practical accomplishment in everyday settings.

In this chapter, we hope to orientate the reader to how the focal research programme, which we termed *MDTsInAction*, developed. We then explore briefly the global concern to enhance interprofessional working and the UK manifestation of this as multidisciplinary teams (MDTs). A literature review of the effects of communication failures in health care is then presented, identifying some of the foundational concerns for this research programme. Finally, the broad aims and methods of the research programme are included before introducing the remainder of the book.

The Development of the *MDTsInAction* Research Programme

The *MDTsInAction* research programme was developed within Plymouth University Clinical Psychology Training Programme. The lead researcher, CS, as a research tutor participated in a number of discussions in teaching groups, reading groups, service user groups and with clinicians around mental health care of different forms. The conversations included hearing the frustrations of service users that decisions seemed to be made that were "beyond their control" (see Chapter 13). Service users told us that one member of staff did not seem to know what another was doing or had told them. They cited examples of how it had been very difficult for them to get input or support from different practitioners, the very reason that interprofessional care exists.

Discussions with staff and clinical psychology trainees revealed frustrations in knowing how to be heard in team meetings, perceived difficulties with power hierarchies, and difficulties in expressing and actioning service user perspectives. The staff and trainees seemed frustrated that they were being, or had been, trained to work in teams together, but that these approaches were idealised and did not match the complexities of actual team working (see Chapter 2). Within the local clinical psychology training programme, trainees noticed that they were trained mainly in therapeutic interventions such as family therapy, which promotes good local relationships within families, and yet, some of these ideas did not seem to be more widely understood within team meetings.

At this same time, there were other new changes occurring both locally and nationally in the UK, where services were increasingly adapting to use what the NHS termed multidisciplinary teams to form diagnoses together (NHS England, 2014), for example in memory clinic and neurodevelopmental services. These new clinic-type approaches necessitated even more a form of joint working between clinicians, taking the entirety of the responsibility away from the medically trained professional (see discussion of creeping genericism in Chapters 2 and 10). Alongside this were moves within the professions of clinical psychology and mental health to develop the notion of team formulation (Johnstone & Boyle, 2018). Formulation has been evolving in clinical psychology for at least 20 years as a way of understanding mental well-being for service users that considers the multiple different factors that are involved in maintaining behaviours that are distressing (Johnstone & Dallos, 2014). Team formulation is now evolving, emphasising how these "assessments" of need could be enhanced through multiple professionals engaging in formulation together (See Chapter 7). A research question which follows on from these developments is to understand exactly how teams of professionals jointly accomplish their formulation of people's problems.

Although there have been attempts to answer this research question, these attempts have frequently relied on qualitative methodologies in which interviewees provide a retrospective account of their experiences or on ethnographic approaches which rely on participant observation of teams in action. These approaches do not accurately capture the moment-to-moment engagement of team members with one another and are subject to a range of epistemological limitations. Our own solution to understanding how teams work is to examine team interactions at a micro-level of detail (see Chapter 2). Over the last 50 years, there has been significant development in discursive methods so that we are now better able to examine in detail how social interaction is organised and to explore how meanings are generated and changed. Studies in this vein were initiated by the work of Harvey Sacks in the 1970s and have gradually moved from analyses of phone calls to include face-to-face interactions and institutional contexts. This approach to studying social interaction generally goes under the title conversation analysis (Sidnell, 2010). The availability of these methods offered the unique possibility of examining how face-to-face team interactions actually work. The challenge, however, was that no one had really done this before—there was not a clear model for how this would work, and the development of small studies into larger ones had limited protocols.

Multidisciplinary Team (MDT) Meetings as a Focal Research Context

The main literature that merges with this understanding of team working is that on interprofessional education (IPE) and interprofessional working (IPW). In 2013, the World Health Organisation (WHO) presented a global framework for action on interprofessional education and collaborative practice, including a call for action. They highlight the necessity of multiple perspectives coming together to enhance patient care. This emphasis comes alongside the development of organisations such as CAIPE (Collaborative for the Advancement of InterProfessional Education) and Plaintree—an organisation devoted to person-centred care.

The current research programme focused on MDT working as this was the term used in the local UK context. Multidisciplinary teams will be defined as composed of members from different healthcare professions with specialised skills and expertise. We will explore some of the different contexts of MDTs, differences in their composition, organisation and function in different healthcare services and structures internationally, throughout this book. We will explore their particular value in supporting people with complex mental health or related needs, and how they can generate individual treatment plans based on "best practice", and enable more immediate care from different professionals, avoiding complex and lengthy referrals (Borril et al., 2001; Fox et al., 2018; Iliffe, 2008; Payne, 2000). However, the book also covers some of the challenges inherent within MDT meetings. Notably, this book focuses only on those MDT meetings where service users (or their carers) are not present (see Chapter 3). We considered this as important, particularly given that service user involvement is constantly emphasised as important in all decisions (for example the WHO's (2015) emphasis on patient voice and the UK's Department of Health (2012) paper "No decision about me without me" (DoH, 2012)). These meetings, however, include many decisions made, where for many logistical reasons service users can not be present, such as whether a person should be accepted to a service, or to review their quality of care. The meetings therefore challenge at some level a value-based health care, which emphasises total involvement of services. However, we consider that overlooking these meetings would not present an honest picture of the real context of mental health care services, and the challenges that clinicians, service users and carers experience around service user involvement and advocacy.

The UK's focus on the importance of MDTs has evolved in an attempt to address care failures in the UK. Reports such as the Winterbourne Report (DoH, 2012) and the Care Act (DoH, 2014) illustrate "top down" attempts to advocate for improved communication at different levels, including within MDT meetings, in order to avoid future cases of neglect. They describe how to make changes and collaborate from the "outside" looking in onto health care. Indeed, they attempt to address how organisational cultures might at least in part contribute to the challenges of joined-up communication. However, we offer a conversation analytic approach (CA) as a way of understanding social organisation from the minutia of interactions, a "bottom up" approach to identifying institutional practices that might also serve as a focus for making changes in organisational culture (See Chapter 2). This opens the possibility of examining how the social organisation of MDTs constrains talk so that information is not presented in the meeting, or is presented in certain ways. We suggest that although healthcare team research has sought to improve team communications through refining understandings of concepts such as collaboration (D'Amour, Goulet, Labadie, Martín-Rodriguez, & Pineault, 2008) and developing descriptive models of teamwork (Mosser & Begun, 2013), more consideration needs to be given to how clinicians actually talk to each other in everyday contexts such as MDT meetings. Therefore, we argue for a focus on the MDT meeting as it is enacted, the place where many decisions are made, but where service users might not be present. We suggest this has implications beyond examining the specific settings of mental health care explored within this book. We argue that a language-aware approach has wider implications for reflecting on how to change and develop mental healthcare cultures to achieve better communication and greater focus on service user experience.

The Challenges of Poor Communication

In order to identify some of the main concerns for the *MDTsInAction* research programme, we conducted a range of literature searches. Most significantly, we attempted to identify what the effects of poor communication can be. Communication difficulties generally between professionals in healthcare settings have been identified as a key causal element of preventable disability or death across the globe (Chassin & Becher, 2002; Wilson et al., 1995). Within the UK, there have been a number of serious incidents resulting in significant consequences for service users, including severe neglect, abuse and a number of unnecessary deaths (Department of Health, 2012; The Mid Staffordshire Foundation Inquiry, 2013). These reports identified that communication failings appeared to be a consistent contributing factor to serious incidents. The Francis Report into Mid Staffordshire NHS Foundation Trust highlights, "This situation was exacerbated by a lack of effective communication across the healthcare system in sharing information and concerns. Organisations relied on others to keep them informed rather than actively seeking and sharing intelligence. At the heart of the failure was a lack of openness, transparency and candour in the information emanating from the Trust and over-reliance on that information by others" (The Mid Staffordshire Foundation Inquiry, 2013, p. 64).

Interestingly, the Francis Inquiry report also identified that "There was insufficient consideration given to the importance of communication with regulatory and supervisory bodies in order to ensure that relevant information pertinent to patient safety was properly disseminated, discussed and appropriate action considered" (The Mid Staffordshire Foundation Inquiry, 2013, p. 60). This highlights that although communication within healthcare settings is increasingly becoming an important factor to consider when accessing how care is provided, historically there has been little focus placed upon this.

Our literature review, then, sought to examine what research has been done concerning poor communication and its effects. A systematic search of the literature was conducted on 26 August 2016 using

PsycINFO; Medline EBSCOhost; Cochrane; and SocINDEX. With the search terms: Communication AND ("Poor" OR "lack of") AND ("multidisciplinary" OR "multi professional" OR "interdisciplinary" OR "Inter-professional") AND ("impact" OR "consequences" OR "Experiences") AND ("service user" OR "patient" OR "client") AND "Healthcare".

The abstracts of each article were then scrutinised, resulting in 6 articles that were written in English and examined professional communication within teams and the consequence to service users. Quality was assessed using the Critical Appraisal Skills Programme (CASP, 2014), and were all considered high quality (Table 1.1). Six articles were included in the review: Ahluwalia, Bekelman, Huynh, Prendergast, and Shreve (2015), Davis, Devoe, Kansagara, Nicolaidis, and Englander (2012), Nagpal et al. (2012), Redfern, Brown, and Vincent (2009), Sutcliffe, Lewton, and Ronsenthal (2004), and Williams et al. (2007), based on physical and medical healthcare settings (Summarised in Table 1.2). The review sought to answer:

1. *What does the literature indicate about what may happen when communication is poor within healthcare teams?* and
2. *What are the consequences for the service user?*

The main findings are summarised here.

Definition Challenges. There was little consistency in terms of how poor communication was described—potentially leading to difficulties for research in terms of considering whether the same phenomenon is being identified. Terms included "communication difficulties", "miscommunication" (Sutcliffe et al., 2004); "distorted or inhibited communication"; "information transfer and communication errors" (Williams et al., 2007); "failure modes" (Redfern et al., 2009); "communication failures and vulnerabilities" (Nagpal et al., 2012); and "poor multidisciplinary communication" and "Ineffective communication" (Ahluwalia et al., 2015; Davis et al., 2012). The papers included letters,

Table 1.1 CASP ratings for literature review on poor communication

CASP	Ahluwalia et al. (2015)	Davis et al. (2012)	Nagpal et al. (2012)	Redfern et al. (2009)	Sutcliffe et al. (2004)	Williams et al. (2007)
Clear statement of aims?	Yes	Yes	Yes	Yes	Yes	Yes
Appropriate qualitative methodology?	Yes	Yes	Yes	Yes	Yes	Can't tell
Was the research design appropriate for addressing the aims?	Yes	Yes	Yes	Yes	Yes	Yes
Was the recruitment strategy appropriate to suit the aims of the research?	Yes	Yes	Yes	Yes	Yes	Yes
Was the data collected in a way that addressed the research issue?	Yes	Yes	Yes	Yes	Yes	Yes
Has the relationship between participant and researcher been adequately considered?	No	No	Can't tell	No	Can't tell	No
Have ethical issues been taken into consideration?	Can't tell	Yes	Yes	Can't tell	Yes	Yes
Was the data analysis sufficiently rigorous?	Yes	Yes	Yes	Yes	Yes	Yes
Is there a clear statement of findings?	Yes	Yes	Yes	Yes	Yes	Yes
How valuable is the research?	Yes	Yes	Yes	Yes	Yes	Yes
Total CASP rating	8	9	9	8	9	8

Table 1.2 A summary of the articles selected for the literature review

Author(s) and title	Aim of study	Sample	Method	Main findings	CASP rating
K. M. Sutcliffe et al. (2004). Communication failures: An insidious contributor to medical mishaps	To describe how communication failures contribute to many medical mishaps	26 residents stratified by medical specialty, year of residency and gender were randomly selected from a population of 85 residents at a 600-bed U.S. teaching hospital	The study consisted of individual semi-structured face-to-face interviews. An inductive case analysis was used	Residents reported a total of 70 mishap incidents. Aspects of "communication" and "patient management" were the two most commonly cited contributing factors. Residents described themselves as embedded in a complex network of relationships. Recurring patterns of communication difficulties occur within these relationships and appear to be associated with the occurrence of medical mishaps	9

(continued)

Table 1.2 (continued)

Author(s) and title	Aim of study	Sample	Method	Main findings	CASP rating
R. G. Williams et al. (2007) Surgeon information transfer and communication: Factors affecting quality and efficiency of inpatient care	To determine the nature of surgeon information transfer and communication (ITC) errors that lead to adverse events and near misses. To recommend strategies for minimising or preventing these errors	Semi-structured focus group sessions were conducted with surgical residents (n = 59), general surgery attending physicians (n = 36) and surgical nurses (n = 42) at 5 medical centres in the USA	The data were collected through direct observations, focus groups and a web-based survey. A constant comparative approach was used to identify main classifications	A total of 328 case descriptions and general comments were obtained and classified. Incidents fell into 4 areas: blurred boundaries of responsibility (87 reports), decreased surgeon familiarity with patients (123 reports), diversion of surgeon attention (31 reports) and distorted or inhibited communication (67 reports). Results were subdivided into 30 contributing factors (e.g. shift change, location change and number of providers). Consequences of ITC lapses included delays in patient care (77% of cases), wasted surgeon/staff time (48%) and serious adverse patient consequences (31%). Twelve principles and 5 institutional habit changes are recommended to guide ITCP re-engineering	8

(continued)

Table 1.2 (continued)

Author(s) and title	Aim of study	Sample	Method	Main findings	CASP rating
E. Redfern et al. (2009). Identifying vulnerabilities in communication in the emergency department	To describe the investigation of communication processes within the emergency department, identify points of vulnerability and guide improvement strategies	All emergency department staff who work at a teaching hospital in London. The pathway of ten "stable" patients was followed. 16 members of the emergency team were interviewed (doctors $n = 7$, nurses $n = 6$; emergency team assistant $n = 1$; porter $n = 1$; receptionist $n = 1$)	A failure mode effects analysis which consists of individual structured interviews was used	A minimum of 19 communication events occurred per patient; all of these events were found to have failure modes which could compromise patient safety. The use of failure mode effects analysis allows members of the MDT to uncover the problem within the system and design counter-measures to improve patient safety	8

(continued)

Table 1.2 (continued)

Author(s) and title	Aim of study	Sample	Method	Main findings	CASP rating
K. Nagpal et al. (2012). Failures in communication and information transfer across the surgical care pathway: Interview study	To explore the communication and information transfer failures across the entire surgical care pathway	18 members of the multidisciplinary team (surgeons $n = 7$; anaesthetists $n = 5$ and nurses $n = 6$) in an acute national health service trust within the UK	Individual semi-structured interviews were conducted. A emergent theme analysis was used	Lack of communication between anaesthetists and surgeons was the most common problem. Incomplete handover from the ward to the theatre and theatre to recovery was other key problems. Work environment, lack of protocols and primitive forms of information transfer were reported as the most common causes of failures. Participants reported that these failures led to increased morbidity and mortality. Healthcare staff were strongly supportive of the view that standardisation and systematisation of communication processes were essential to improve patient safety	9

(continued)

Table 1.2 (continued)

Author(s) and title	Aim of study	Sample	Method	Main findings	CASP rating
M. M. Davis et al. (2012). "Did I do as best as the system would let me?" Healthcare professional views on hospital to home care transitions	To understand care transitions from the perspective of diverse healthcare professionals and identify recommendations for process improvement	75 healthcare professionals and administrators from both inpatient ($n=25$) and outpatient ($n=13$) setting, 12 covered both settings, within health services in the USA	13 focus groups and 2 in-depth interviews with participants. A thematic analysis was used to identify emergent themes and a cross-case comparative analysis to describe variation by participant role and setting	Poor transitional care reflected healthcare system fragmentation, limiting the ability of healthcare professionals to provide optimal patient care. Lack of standardised processes, poor MDT communication within the hospital and fragmented communication across the settings led to chaotic, unsystematic transitions, poor patient outcomes, and feelings of futility and dissatisfaction among providers. Patients with complex psychosocial needs were especially vulnerable during care transitions. Recommended changes to improve transitional care included improving MDT hospital rounds, clarifying accountability as patients move across settings, standardising discharge processes and providing additional medical staff training	9

(continued)

Table 1.2 (continued)

Author(s) and title	Aim of study	Sample	Method	Main findings	CASP rating
S. C. Ahluwalia et al. (2015). Barriers and strategies to an iterative model of advance care planning communication	Identifying veteran affair provider's perspectives on barriers and strategies for using an iterative model of advanced care planning. Characterise barriers and strategies for realising an interactive model of advanced care planning patient-provider communication	20 providers (professionals: physicians (13); nursing (3); social work (2); chaplaincy (2) from veterans affair medical centre in America	2 multidisciplinary team focus groups and 3 semi-structured interviews were conducted. Thematic analysis was employed to identify salient themes	Barriers included variations among providers in approaches to advanced care planning, lack of useful information about patient value to guide decision-making and ineffective communication between providers across settings. Strategies included eliciting patient values rather than specific treatment choices and an increased role of primary care advances in care planning processes	8

notes and telephone conversations, not just meetings, as none of the studies focused solely on team meetings. Common communication problems were identified as: "lack of information" and "misinterpretation" (Sutcliffe et al., 2004, p. 188); "lost information and time delays" (Redfern et al., 2009, p. 656). One article noted that the quality of information was being compromised when sent via methods other than face to face (Williams et al., 2007).

Service User Effects. Effects on service users included patient management, diagnosis and extreme treatment errors including "..near misses to invasive treatments being carried out wrongly (a chest tube being inserted in the wrong side of a patient)" (Sutcliffe et al., 2004, p. 188), or cancelled operations (Nagpel et al., 2012). Delays in service user care were related to communication; 77% of all days delayed were related to mortality and serious morbidity (Williams et al., 2007, p. 164). Redfern et al. (2009, p. 656) identified more general failures such as "poor patient care, loss of patient information, delays and inefficiency". Papers frequently cited increased length of hospital stay (Nagpel et al., 2012) and medication errors (Davis et al., 2012). Finally, Ahluwalia et al. (2015) observed that poor staff communication led to a lack of person-centredness, as in-depth information about how people wanted to be cared for at the end of their lives was not considered.

Organisation Effects. The review highlighted that poor communication affects professionals and the provider as well as service users. Resources and staff time were frequently wasted (Davis et al. 2012; Nagpal et al., 2012; Redfern et al., 2009; Sutcliffe et al., 2004; Williams et al., 2007). Redfern et al. (2009) highlighted how this lengthens inpatient stays before transfer to community settings. Nagpal et al. (2012) stress the financial impact of these effects.

Staff Effects. Other staff effects include questioning the reputation, and decreased credibility, of professionals and organisations (Williams et al., 2007). These compound factors also affected staff happiness and morale (Davis et al., 2012; Nagpal et al., 2012; Williams et al., 2007). Davies et al. (2012) identified that poor communication within teams "profoundly affects MDT provider job satisfaction" (p. 1654). Ahluwalia et al. (2015) identified that staff expressed frustration when there is an absence or inaccessibility of information, such as the patients' healthcare values and goals, due to poor communication between professionals. This can overall affect decision-making and the care the team provides. More specifically the lack of communication between professions was noted to cause "role confusion" or members of the team "being left out of decision-making" (Davis et al., 2012, p. 1653), which not only has an impact on professionals but may also have an impact on the quality of care delivered.

Hierarchy and Profession Effects. The effects of hierarchy were a further theme. Sutcliffe et al. (2004) and Williams et al. (2007) identified that junior staff often expressed fears of appearing incompetent to superiors and therefore hesitated to communicate information as they wanted to maintain a favourable impression. This was fuelled by junior staff fearing that they may be unnecessarily bothering senior staff. Nagpal et al. (2012) also identified that there was a "hierarchical obstruction to the flow of information", and often junior staff were not sufficiently empowered to play an active role, which ultimately contributed to information transfer and communication failures. Williams et al. (2007) further noted that blurred boundaries of responsibility between professionals could result in "unclear delegation of responsibility" (Williams et al., 2007, p. 161), which contributed to miscommunication between professionals. Williams et al. (2007) also described how assumptions made by professionals about the knowledge, skills or understanding of other professionals can influence the quantity and quality of information communicated.

Face-to-Face Communication. These profound effects of poor communication to the detriment of both service users and staff were frequently accounted for in research by poor interprofessional skills. Davis et al. (2012) commented on some of the consequences when there is a reduction in face-to-face communication and interaction between professionals. For example, electronic medical record systems being relied upon more frequently as a way to communicate information have resulted in unintended negative consequences on interpersonal communication. One participant commented, "… discharge can happen without us ever actually speaking to doctors" (Davis et al., 2012, p. 1653). Ahluwalia et al. (2015) also described, "… one of the biggest barriers is we're so big as an institution and so siloed in terms of structure that we don't know each other like we used to. It's not easy to call someone you don't know and you're afraid you're interrupting them" (Ahluwalia et al., 2015, p. 819). Sutcliffe et al. (2004) further added that the non-verbal communication between staff also contributed to how much information was shared between staff during conversations. Participants commented on how this was influenced by how "nice" or "aggressive" colleagues appeared (p. 192). Nagpal et al. (2012) also described how primitive forms of information, such as based on poorly designed and completed forms, reduced the quality of information being transferred between professionals.

In summary, this review of poor communication in healthcare teams raises several key issues that the *MDTsInAction* programme should consider. First, the ambiguity in identifying what "poor" communication is, and therefore potentially also what good communication might be. This ambiguity further emphasised the value of a conversation analytic/discursive psychology approach that is able to reveal and describe interactional practices in detail. Rather than imposing a judgement, it enables us to heighten our and others' awareness (see Chapters 14 and 15) of how talk has an effect. The review highlights the significant effects for service users, though unfortunately there were less clear examples of the effects of mental health. It also emphasises the organisational level of effects—in terms of reputation and effectiveness, the effects for staff in terms of potential burnout and difficulties, and effects of significant organisational factors such as power hierarchies. Significantly for our research programme was the emphasis in the review on the essential nature of face-to-face interactions. These themes, around how organisational and emotional factors influence team meetings, how clinical work is achieved, and how service users are affected, are explored in the different sections of the book.

Aims and Methods of the *MDTsInAction* Research Programme

The *MDTsInAction* research programme sought to open up a new pathway to understanding how to study mental healthcare team working contexts. It specifically sought to find ways to understand how face-to-face communications work, given that this seems to be a key area that is problematic in the literature, and to develop ways of improving this communication. We wanted to explore how people enact team working and to develop useful and relevant implications for practice.

The *MDTsInAction* research project developed to include consultation and projects completed by a range of trained and trainee clinical psychologists, carers, service users, academics, undergraduates and masters students. As a core group, we included psychologists, a nurse, social scientists and service users. The project began in 2013 and is ongoing in 2018. Twelve of the projects from the programme are included in this book. The 12 different projects can be divided into three areas, those focused on: clinical, organisational or team activities. Clinical activities included concerns such as developing team formulations; organisational activities were around business meetings and the structure of meetings; and team activities included interpersonal support and professional development. We found, as we delved into the data, that there were numerous foci that could have guided the project, and these were iteratively developed throughout the project.

The main focus of the study was on teams working with people with mental health needs. This focus was related to the professional interests of the research team. We have included MDTs from specialities including: adult mental health, neurodevelopment, dementia care, intellectual disabilities, pain care teams and early intervention psychosis. We hope that this diversity strengthens the research in allowing us to illustrate the multiple applications of the approaches, exploring the different uses of language in interaction that occur in these different specialities. Within these specialities, we have also included different types of MDTs that are shaped in different ways by the services that they are embedded in. For example, some met weekly, some less and some more. Some included large numbers (18), others smaller (7–10) of participants. We recorded as many meetings as we could including business meetings, allocations meetings (where service users were allocated to services), case review meetings and peer review meetings. We hope that this also reflects some of the very different compositions of MDTs that are prevalent within health care, and how these different structures affect the different interactions that are enacted.

The Development of a Conversation Analytic Project

This book not only reports the findings from the *MDTsInAction* research programme, it also seeks to illustrate the way in which a conversation analytic project was developed—from its very beginnings into a mature and impactful research programme. Earlier in this chapter, we have described how the focal research question of this project emerged from discussions with students, colleagues, service users and healthcare professionals. The principal investigators of this project already had a knowledge and understanding of conversation analysis and discursive psychology, and thereby could discern how these methodologies offered both a unique insight into the practical accomplishment of multidisciplinary team meetings and a partnership with professionals in developing their understanding and skills in achieving their professional aims through MDTs. In pursuing these twin facets of the project, we were mindful that we had to maintain an academic thoroughness in our analysis of MDT meetings without losing sight of the original clinical concerns which had animated the project in the first place.

There are a number of ways in which the practical development of this project is discernible in the chapters which follow. The majority of those who have contributed to this book undertook the research as the major dissertation for their doctoral programme in clinical psychology. Through seminar discussions and teaching sessions, an important learning point was an increased sensitivity to language. These students were already acutely aware of the power that language has to label, stigmatise, demean and also liberate those who use or are the recipients of others' talk. What was necessary was for them to develop an understanding of how language in use worked, as Harvey Sacks put it how "the machineries of talk" operated. Through teaching but also importantly the use of data sessions with CARP (our local CA research group), we inducted these students into the principles and foundational concepts of conversation analysis and discursive psychology. We see how a growing understanding of CA/DP principles allowed these tyro-researchers to develop a detailed understanding and insight into practices which professional staff utilised to accomplish their aims of gaining a multiprofessional input into the cases they brought to the MDTs. For example, Parish (Chapter 8) identifies how meeting participants engage in displays of uncertainty and news receipts as methodical ways of opening up particular cases for input from other professionals.

However, not all followed a strict adherence to the CA/DP model. Others chose a critical discursive psychology route, and the findings which emerged from that route (see Chapter 13) were invaluable in providing evidence of not just health professionals' concerns about whether MDTs were fit for purpose but also of service users' commensurate concerns. This part of the research programme led directly to a very important research question, namely how absent service users were represented in meetings and concomitantly how health professionals advocated for their users.

Another facet of the research programme which emerges strongly through many chapters is the ethical responsibilities of pursuing a CA/DP approach. Discursive methodologies throw up unique ethical challenges, particularly in that obtaining video or audio recordings of real meetings is a necessary part of the analytic procedure. This requirement entails a sensitive engagement with gatekeepers of the organisation (often the ethics committees or research boards) as well as those whose talk and actions are going to be recorded. These matters are addressed in detail in Chapter 3 but are also referred to in many other of the empirical chapters. For example, Aikman (Chapter 6) and Parish (Chapter 8) refer to using "bracketing interviews" as a methodological amendment to a strict CA approach which allowed them to feel confident that their analyses were commensurate with the lived experiences of their research participants. Bracketing interviews are undertaken before data collection and during the data analysis stage (Rolls & Relf, 2006). This is a process in which one acknowledges, or "brackets off", subjective assumptions in an attempt to reduce the impact of these in the analysis. For this, the researcher was interviewed by a colleague about the project, specifically questioning about assumptions, feelings or personal connections to the topic. These interviews were recorded and transcribed, so they could be referred back at set times points, such as after the initial data analysis. For the researchers, they also provided an insight into the processes of developing an interpretation of the data.

These accounts of the specific research projects throw into sharp relief how this sort of research programme has to be a meaningful partnership if it is to yield findings of value both for the broader academic community and for those working every day in the healthcare and social care professions. One of the unique ways in which this partnership was developed was through engaging the professional staff in joint analysis sessions (see Chapter 14).

Finally, this research programme always set out to be an applied CA programme. Antaki (2011) has identified six kinds of application of conversation analytic research. These six are summarised as: foundational, social problem oriented, communicational, diagnostic, institutional and interventionist. For many of the authors, there were elements of all six kinds of application running through their research, and in order to achieve a satisfactory level of application, they often adapted their CA methodology to achieve meaningful application in partnership with their research participants (see above). One important vehicle for application which became a key part of the research programme was the implementation of joint analysis. Having obtained initial data, and having undertaken an initial level of analysis, extracts from the recordings along with transcriptions were taken back to the original participants for further ways of understanding the actions and practices identifiable in the interactions. This facet of the research programme is described in detail in Chapter 14.

Organisation of the Book

In order to meet the research questions raised by the literature review and the problem of communication in health care, and specifically in mental health care, this book is organised into 5 separate sections.

In the first section, we will examine the development of the research methods. We have very briefly introduced discursive methods in this chapter, but we will examine these further and elaborate on how these methods are able to shed light on the mental healthcare team. In the second section, we focus on the broad functions of team meetings. We present a discursive model of how meetings can be conceptualised and of how the different concerns of the participants are displayed in the meeting interactions. Thirdly, we examine some of the clinical applications of these meetings—how team formulations might operate, trying to draw out what this can look like in a team, and what the key points in formulation are. Next, we examine in more detail how service user experiences are represented, including a chapter that has been written by service users about staff, and how advocacy occurs within team meetings. Finally, we include a section on the interventions arising from the research that we have done—we detail how joint analysis might work, and its utility, rather uniquely with a non-conversation analysis group, and then outline our suggestion for a training programme based on this innovative approach to understanding communication.

In sum, we would like to be able to argue that this research programme has made a contribution to the body of knowledge within the discipline of conversation analysis. It has had a positive impact on the healthcare and social care professionals who participated in the research and their organisational conduct. It has also contributed to the values of the authors who graduated as clinical psychologists particularly in terms of their ability to act as reflective practitioners.

References

Ahluwalia, S. C., Bekelman, D. B., Huynh, A. K., Prendergast, T. J., Shreve, S., & Lorenz, K. A. (2015). Barriers and strategies to an iterative model of advance care planning communication. *The American Journal of Hospice & Palliative Care, 32*(8), 817–823. https://doi.org/10.1177/1049909114541513.

Antaki, C. (2011). Six kinds of applied conversation analysis. In C. Antaki (Ed.), *Applied conversation analysis: Intervention and change in institutional talk*. Basingstoke: Palgrave Macmillan.

Borrill, C. S., Carletta, J., Carter, A. J., Dawson, J. F., Garrod, S. Rees, A., …, West, M. A. (2001). *The effectiveness of health care teams in the National Health Service*. Aston University. Retrieved on 10 May 2016 from http:// homepages.inf.ed.ac.uk/jeanc/DOH-final-report.pdf.

CASP Checklists. (2014). *Critical Appraisal Skills Programme*. Retrieved 17 October 2016 from http://media.wix.com/ugd/dded87_29c5b002d99342f-788c6ac670e49f274.pdf.

Chassin, M. R., & Becher, E. C. (2002). The wrong patient. *Annals of Internal Medicine, 136*, 826–833.

Chong, W. W., Aslani, P., & Chen, T. F. (2013). Multiple perspectives on shared decision-making and interprofessional collaboration in mental healthcare. *Journal of Interprofessional Care, 27*(3), 223–230. https://doi.org /10.3109/13561820.2013.767225.

D'Amour, D., Goulet, L., Labadie, J.-F., Martín-Rodriguez, L. S., & Pineault, R. (2008). A model and typology of collaboration between professionals in healthcare organizations. *BMC Health Services Research 2008, 8*, 188. https://doi.org/10.1186/1472-6963-8-188.

Davis, M. M., Devoe, M., Kansagara, D., Nicolaidis, C., & Englander, H. (2012). "Did I do as best as the system would let me?" Healthcare professional views on hospital to home care transitions. *Journal of General Internal Medicine, 27*(12), 1649–1656. https://doi.org/10.1007/ s11606-012-2169-3.

Department of Health (DoH). (2012). *Winterbourne view hospital: Department of health review and response*. Retrieved from https:// www.gov.uk/government/publications/winterbourne-view-hospital-department-of-health-review-and-response.

Department of Health (DoH). (2013). *The report of the Mid Staffordshire NHS Foundation Trust public inquiry*. Retrieved from: https://www.gov.uk/government/uploads/system/uploads/attachment_data/file/279124/0947.pdf.

Department of Health. (2014). *The care act*. London: Department of Health.

Fox, L., Onders, R., Hermansen-Kobulnicky, C. J., Nguyen, T.-N., Myran, L., Linn, B., & Hornecker, J. (2018). Teaching interprofessional teamwork skills to health professional students: A scoping review. *Journal of Interprofessional Care, 32*(2), 127–135. https://doi.org/10.1080/13561820. 2017.1399868

Iliffe, S. (2008). Myths and realities in multidisciplinary team-working. *London Journal of Primary Care, 1*(2), 100–102.

Johnston, L., & Dallos, R. (2014). *Formulation in psychology and psychotherapy: Making sense of people's problems* (2nd ed.). Hove: Routledge.

Johnstone, L., & Boyle, M., with Cromby, J., Dillon, J., Harper, D., Kinderman, P., Longden, E., Pilgrim, D., & Read, J. (2018). *The power threat meaning framework: Towards the identification of patterns in emotional distress, unusual experiences and troubled or troubling behaviour, as an alternative to functional psychiatric diagnosis.* Leicester: British Psychological Society.

Mosser, G., & Begun, J. W. (2013). *Understanding teamwork in health care.* New York: McGraw Hill Professional.

Nagpal, K., Arora, S., Vats, A., Wong, H. W., Sevdalis, N., Vincent, C., & Moorthy, K. (2012). Failures in communication and information transfer across the surgical care pathway: Interview study. *British Medical Journal of Quality & Safety, 21*(10), 843–849.

National Health Service (NHS) England. (2014). *MDT Development—Working towards an effective multidisciplinary/multiagency team.* Retrieved from https://www.england.nhs.uk/wp-content/uploads/2015/01/mdt-dev-guid-flat-fin.pdf.

Payne, M. (2000). *Teamwork in multiprofessional care.* Basingstoke: Palgrave.

Redfern, E., Brown, R., & Vincent, C. A. (2009). Identifying vulnerabilities in communication in the emergency department. *Emergency Medicine Journal: EMJ, 26*(9), 653–657. https://doi.org/10.1136/emj.2008.065318.

Rolls, L., & Relf, M. (2006). Bracketing interviews: Addressing methodological challenges in qualitative interviewing in bereavement and palliative care. *Mortality, 11,* 286–305.

Sidnell, J. (2010). *Conversation analysis: An introduction.* Chichester: Wiley-Blackwell.

Sutcliffe, K. M., Lewton, E., & Rosenthal, M. M. (2004). Communication failures: An insidious contributor to medical mishaps. *Academic Medicine, 79,* 186–194.

Williams, R. G., Silverman, R., Schwind, C., Fortune, M. D., Sutyak, M. D., Horvath, K., ..., Dunnington, G. L., (2007). Surgeon information transfer and communication: Factors affecting quality and efficiency of inpatient care. *Ann Surg, 245,* 159e69.

Wilson, R. M., Runciman, W. B., Gibberd, R. W., Harrison, B. T., Newby, L., & Hamilton, J. D. (1995). The quality in Australian health care study. *Medical Journal of Australia, 63,* 458–471.

World Health Organisation. (2013). *Framework for action on interprofessional education and collaboration.* Geneva: The World Health Organisation.

World Health Organisation. (2015). *People-centred health systems in the WHO European region: Voices of patients and carers.* Geneva, Switzerland: The World Health Organisation.

Part I

Researching Multi-disciplinary Teams Using a Language Based Perspective

2

Inside the Meeting: Discursive Approaches as a Framework for Understanding Multidisciplinary Team Meetings

Timothy Auburn, Cordet Smart and Madeleine Tremblett

Background

In 2001, Drew, Chatwin and Collins noted that '*At the very heart of the delivery of health-care services lie the interactions between medical staff and patients*'. This arena of interaction they further note is key for accurate diagnosis, gaining the cooperation of patients to comply with treatment plans as well as achieving patient satisfaction. The sentiments of this observation can be expanded to teams of health and social care professionals: *at the very heart of the delivery of health care services lie the interactions between health care professionals themselves.*

T. Auburn (✉) · C. Smart · M. Tremblett
School of Psychology, University of Plymouth, Plymouth, UK
e-mail: T.Auburn@plymouth.ac.uk

C. Smart
e-mail: cordet.smart@plymouth.ac.uk

M. Tremblett
e-mail: madeleine.tremblett@plymouth.ac.uk

© The Author(s) 2018
C. Smart and T. Auburn (eds.), *Interprofessional Care and Mental Health*,
The Language of Mental Health, https://doi.org/10.1007/978-3-319-98228-1_2

The interaction between healthcare professionals through teamworking is increasingly regarded as essential to the delivery of effective patient-centred health and social care (see Chapter 1). This focus has come about over several decades, occasioned by a number of factors: the increasing complexity of and multidisciplinarity underlying healthcare decisions (Bokhour, 2006; Reeves, Lewin, Espin, & Zwarenstein, 2010); the increasing overlap between health and social care and the need to deliver care in a different way (D'Amour, Goulet, Labadie, Rodriguez, & Pineault, 2008; Health and Social Care Act, 2012); and the emergence of several scandals in England, UK, where care was found to be woefully inadequate in part through lack of communication between different professionals (e.g. Francis Report, 2013, recommendation 237). These and other factors have led policymakers towards the implementation of interprofessional care, whereby health and social care professionals from different backgrounds are expected to collaborate in the decisions which bear upon the treatment and care of individual patients. In so doing, the expectation is that the quality of patient care will improve and that overload and other stresses upon professional staff will reduce (see Chapter 6).

Interprofessional care requires a degree of collaboration, teamwork or networking (Reeves, Xyrichis, & Zwarenstein, 2018) between professionals with a stake in healthcare decisions. Zwarenstein, Goldman, and Reeves (2009) have defined interprofessional collaboration as follows: '*Interprofessional collaboration (IPC) is the process in which different professional groups work together to positively impact health care. IPC involves a negotiated agreement between professionals which values the expertise and contributions that various healthcare professionals bring to patient care*' (p. 2). Alongside the implementation of systems of interprofessional care, much work has been expended on the factors that determine the quality and fitness for purpose of such systems. Interventions designed to improve the quality of interprofessional care have occurred in three arenas: education for interprofessional care, improvements to interprofessional practice and interventions concerning organisational change (Zwarenstein et al., 2009). The focus of this chapter (and more broadly this book) is on the second of these arenas—interprofessional practice. This focus entails a consideration of how professionals engage directly with one another in pursuing an interprofessional care agenda.

At the core of the practical implementation of interprofessional care is teamwork (D'Amour, Ferrada-Videla, Rodriguez, & Beaulieu, 2005), which in turn is normally operationalised as ward rounds or more usually multidisciplinary team meetings (Field et al., 2010; O'Carroll, McSwiggan, & Campbell, 2016). Though different terminologies have been used to label how a team organises its working—inter, multi and trans (D'Amour et al., 2005), there is a common resemblance across these labels in what is being referred to. Specifically, teamwork encounters are based on different healthcare professionals meeting face-to-face and sharing their knowledge and understanding of a particular patient case. The distinction between these types of teamworking lies largely in the degree of integration and amount of professional autonomy accorded the members of the team (D'Amour et al., 2005). Thus, '... all the terms convey the notion of bridge building between specific disciplines toward a particular goal or goals that require some degree of restructuring of thought and practice' (Deady, 2012, p. 177). The literature has many examples of research into the practice of interprofessional care. Zwarenstein et al. (2009) identified 5 studies for their systematic review of interventions designed to improve interprofessional collaboration. Four of these five were explicitly targeted at the team meetings, either ward rounds or multidisciplinary team meetings. Similarly, Arber (2008) notes that multidisciplinary meetings are a common way of structuring interprofessional relationships in end-of-life care where 'total care' is a key underlying philosophy.

A Problematic Disjuncture

Although the move towards teamwork has been predicated on the aspiration to improve healthcare outcomes, this move has not been without criticism. Several review studies have suggested that MDT meetings have limited measurable effects on patient outcomes (e.g. Pillay et al., 2016; Zwarenstein et al., 2009). One possible explanation is that such outcomes are not achieved because the institutional requirement for MDT meetings does not reflect the contingencies and demands of the everyday working environment of the healthcare professionals. Lewin and Reeves (2011) conducted an ethnographic observation of everyday interprofessional encounters on a busy general and emergency medical directorate in an inner city UK hospital. On the basis of their observation of planned sessions for interprofessional working (i.e. ward rounds and MDT meetings), they argued that effective communication between different professionals was highly constrained and limited. For example, they observed that MDT meetings were of limited value, with doctors rarely attending and thereby little interprofessional communication occurring. Despite the limitations of these formal, planned occasions for interprofessional working, they suggest that both the MDT meetings and the ward rounds be maintained simply as an institutional display of collaboration. They quote one doctor as describing ward rounds as doctors and nurses working in 'parallel' rather than interprofessionally and they note that these planned formal sessions often simply reinforced the established medical hierarchy.

Other studies in which direct observation of interactions between team members was undertaken reinforce this suggestion that there often is a disjuncture between how members and their institutions account for the organisation of work and the practices in which they actually engage (e.g. Wittenberg-Lyles, Oliver, Demiris, & Regehr, 2010). Barnard, Cruice, and Playford (2010) note that in interdisciplinary goal setting meetings with patients present, the professional members of the team showed a concern to transform the goals articulated by the patients into ones which were more commensurate with those which they believed were achievable. Additionally, Bokhour (2006) investigated the implementation of team meetings in a residential dementia care centre; she also interviewed key members of the team. Analysis of the interviews indicated a range of aspirational goals and perspectives on the effectiveness of the care planning meetings; for example, one theme of the interviews was that the meetings should provide 'the best patient care possible' (p. 353). In contrast, her analysis of the conduct of the team meetings themselves allowed her to identify three practices (giving report, writing report and collaborative discussion). Although collaborative discussion is cited as the most frequent practice displayed in the meetings, her example of this practice suggests that it is characterised by disagreement between team members and the dominance of professional medical diagnosis over accounts of members with direct experience of the patient. Bokhour suggests: '*While each of the identified communication practices serves a purpose in the course of the team meetings, the ritualized nature of the process of the meetings has serious consequences for patients. As team members focus primarily on the task of completing a review and an ITP, crucial social and personal information about patients is often excluded*'. In particular, she suggests that the practices of 'giving and writing a report' constrain the participation of other members of the team in planning, thereby excluding relevant patient information.

Where there have been attempts to improve interprofessional communication, the constraints and demands of the organisation have limited the impact of such interventions. Rice et al. (2010) provided a four-step script to professionals working on a general internal medicine ward in a Canadian hospital intended to produce improved communication and collaboration. They note that this intervention was not implemented as intended and failed to produce any improvements in communication or collaboration. They attribute this failure to professional resistance as well as the 'fast-paced, interruptive environment of the ward'.

In addition to evidence of a disjuncture between the aspirational aims of teamworking and its implementation, there is also a range of criticisms relating to its organisational implications. Rice et al. attributed the limited impact of their intervention to professional resistance. It has been argued that such resistance arises from the threat that those assigned to a team perceive from the imposition of an 'evangelistic' managerialist philosophy whose underlying agenda is the increased control of professional staff (Finn, Learmonth, & Reedy, 2010). However, these authors argue that the discourse which is utilised by managers to justify the implementation of teamworking also provides a resource for team members to resist its imposition. They also note the disjuncture between the official rhetoric of teamworking and the discourse that the team members used to characterise their actual working. In one case, team members simply ignored the official rhetoric in favour of a more attractive localised identity ('the girls'); in the other case, the official rhetoric was used to reinforce the professional divisions which it was designed to overcome. This resistance has also been attributed to a sense that the imposition of teamworking amounts to a 'creeping genericism' whereby requiring people to work in teams erodes their sense of professional identity (Brown, Crawford, & Darongkamas, 2000).

Finally, we can note that Reeves et al. (2010) in their extensive review and analysis of interprofessional teamwork hint at this disjuncture problem:

> For us, the inadequate progress in developing a deeper understanding of teamwork is, in part, a result of many teamwork texts and papers being based on a priori assumption that teams are a 'good thing', and that they offer a solution to alleviating a number of the ills of health and social care systems. While there is an intuitive appeal in this view, its consequence is that few authors have drilled down to the empirical, conceptual and theoretical bedrock upon which teamwork rests. (p. 1)

Approaches to Understanding Teamworking

There has been a burgeoning literature on interprofessional working and in particular on meetings as the site where interprofessional working is most often implemented. A common evaluation of these studies is that: '*They do not help us understand what transpires in the working lives of a group of collaborating professionals or the nature of their interactional dynamics*' (D'Amour et al., 2005, p. 126; see also Kuziemsky et al., 2009; Zwarenstein et al., 2009). In addressing this lacuna, there have been a number of studies which employ qualitative methodologies aimed at examining these interactional dynamics. Such methodologies include qualitative interviewing of a purposively selected sample of professionals (e.g. D'Amour et al., 2008), ethnographic observations of teamworking (e.g. Kuziemsky et al., 2009) and discourse analytic methods (e.g. Bélanger et al., 2014). The approach advocated in this book is one based on conversation analysis (CA) (Sacks, 1992; Sidnell, 2010; Sidnell & Stivers, 2013) and its more recent extension discursive psychology (DP) (Edwards & Potter, 1992, 2005; Wiggins, 2017).

The basis of both these approaches (CA/DP) is to describe and thereby understand the organisation of social encounters drawing upon a detailed examination of the sequences of talk recorded in the setting in which they occur. They are methodologies which can be applied to both informal interactions and formal, institutional interactions.

The assumption of these approaches is that it is through the fine details of talk and its accompanying non-verbal features, that social contexts are established and maintained on a moment-to-moment basis (see Chapter 4). Conversation analysis and discursive psychology focus on the organisation of individual turns of talk and what actions are being formed in such turns. Each turn of talk displays, often implicitly, the hearer's understanding of the prior utterance, which in turn forms the basis of their own turn. By monitoring each other's turns of talk, participants provide the basis for establishing a mutual understanding and if necessary repairing that understanding as they go along. This way of conceiving the dynamic flow of talk has been termed 'the architecture of intersubjectivity'. Consequently, no detail is too small to be relevant to the smooth continuation of a conversation. For example, back channel utterances such as 'hm mm' or 'ok' are often designed to ensure that the current speaker maintains the speaking floor.

An example of recent research where an understanding of conversation analytic principles could have informed the study design is Rice et al.'s (2010) intervention which aimed to improve interprofessional communication. In this study, Rice et al. designed a four-step script intervention for the exchange of information 'during all patient related interactions'. The four steps were: (1) providing the speaker's name, (2) stating the speaker's professional role, (3) sharing issues relating to the patient under discussion, and (4) seeking feedback.

At all steps in this script, there are numerous choices about how these actions can be implemented, and each choice will have potentially radically different impacts on the way in which an intersubjective understanding of the patient's case is constructed. As a case in point, Rice et al. suggest that in step 4 feedback can be gained by using prompts such as 'Do you have any concerns?' or 'Is there something else that I should consider?' The work in CA on question design (Heritage, 2010) suggests that these two ways of seeking feedback will normatively elicit very different responses. In the first by using the negative polarity item 'any', the speaker is setting up a normative expectation that the response will be a 'no', the 'preferred' response (see below). In contrast, the use of 'something else' alters the polarity of the question so that the normative response is to respond affirmatively and so provide other concerns.

Heritage, Robinson, Elliot, Beckett, and Wilkes (2007) provided doctors with alternative questions to ask patients at the end of a consultation. When the doctors asked: 'Are there *some* other concerns that you would like to talk about?' over 90% of patients responded with further concerns whereas when the question contained *any* rather than *some* less than 50% responded with further concerns. This illustration points to the need to examine in detail how team meetings (or ward rounds) as the canonical implementation of interprofessional care are organised socially through participants' talk; 'Thus, it is in the local and contextual interactions of participants that organisations are performatively enacted' (Watson & Drew, 2017).

A corollary of this position is to throw some doubt on the value of semi-structured or qualitative research interviewing as being a method fit for the purposes of understanding the interactional dynamics of team meetings (see also Lewin & Reeves, 2011). A particular problem with qualitative research interviews concerns the level of detail that can be elicited about the interaction that occurs in any meeting. By their very nature, qualitative interviews elicit retrospective accounts of the participants' experiences of interprofessional collaboration. Though researchers might take every care to ensure that such accounts are as 'accurate' as possible, they cannot provide the detail required to understand the turn-by-turn organisation of meetings. Such interview accounts are better regarded as the joint accomplishments of the participant *and* researcher in producing a co-constructed version of the participant's prior experiences (Roulston, 2011; Potter & Hepburn, 2005, 2012).

Our preferred approach, therefore, to understanding the nature of teamworking and in particular team meetings, is to adopt methods which allow us to record the actual interaction (audio or preferably video), and transcribing relevant segments of that interaction to a high level of detail (based on Jeffersonian transcription conventions, see Hepburn & Bolden, 2013). Such segments are brought together as collections representing a particular action-oriented practice displayed by the participants themselves. The analyst is then concerned to explicate this practice both how it is organised, what functions it performs and variations in the organisation of this practice which perform then subtly different functions.

The Principles of Conversation Analysis and Discursive Psychology

An 'Etic'/'Emic' Distinction

Conversation analysis and discursive psychology can be characterised as 'emic' approaches to understanding both social interaction and social conduct. 'Emic' approaches contrast with 'etic'; both terms are borrowed from cultural anthropology and before that linguistics. 'Etic' approaches are generally characterised as an outsider's perspective such that the analysis of a culture or group draws upon the analyst's specialist terms and concepts rather than the distinctions and understandings drawn upon by the members themselves. An example of an 'etic' approach within the field of interprofessional care would be Reeves et al. (2010) extensive review of interprofessional teamwork. They employ a range of social science concepts to explain the performance and function of teams; they cluster the factors implicated in teamworking performance under four domains, namely 'relational', 'processual', 'organisational' and 'contextual'. Analysis of teamworking which identifies the factors within each of these domains allows the authors to produce a typology of interprofessional working (teamworking, collaboration, coordination and networking) and suggests which type of working should be matched to particular local settings with their own unique demands.

This approach yields a powerful analysis and one which can feed usefully into a range of policy recommendations and decisions about how to establish interprofessional working. However, we suggest that an 'emic' approach is a necessary preliminary to such 'etic' approaches. 'Emic' approaches are characterised as an 'insider's' perspective. In our case, conversation analysis and discursive psychology provide us with an alternative 'emic' approach, which attends to the concerns and orientations of the participants as displayed in their everyday interactions. Conversation analysis provides us also with a technical vocabulary and set of concepts by which to characterise these participants' orientations. As a consequence, it would not be appropriate to examine team interactions for their performance in terms of their degree of collaboration. Such a move would be to impose an outsider's concept on the participants' activity. Instead, we examine team meetings for the sorts of actions participants themselves display and orient to (see Chapter 4). For example, rather than examining interactions in terms of whether they represent collaboration or not, good communication or not, we wish to examine them for what the participants take themselves to be doing, such as finding a slot to provide relevant information or advocating for a service user.

A good exemplar of this approach is the work of Arber (2008). Arber examined multidisciplinary team meetings in a hospice where palliative care was undertaken. She recorded eight team meetings and then analysed them by first noticing practices which the participants themselves produced in the course of their participation in the meetings. In particular, she noticed that questions were asked disproportionately more frequently by nurses than other members of the teams. Her analysis of the design of these questions and responses they received allowed her to conclude that these questions, often hedged and displaying the delicacy of the medical matters under discussion when a consultant is present, were oriented to the authority and superior medical knowledge of consultants. They were designed, inter alia, to allow nurses to propose medical diagnoses for patient's symptoms without overtly challenging the consultant's medical expertise. Rather than label these encounters as instances of collaboration (which they surely are), through a detailed examination of the design of talk, we can discern the participant's own orientation to the contingencies which the talk is designed to manage.

Ultimately, the distinction between 'etic' and 'emic' is a loose one and there is often an interplay between these two levels of analysis. However, we suggest that by emphasising an 'emic' approach and hence foregrounding participants' own orientations to the work they are undertaking, we will be able to yield a rich and useful body of knowledge which participants can themselves use to develop their practice (see Chapter 14).

Conversation Analysis

Conversation analysis has been defined as: '… an approach within the social sciences that aims to describe, analyse and understand talk as a basic and constitutive feature of human social life' (Sidnell, 2010, p. 1).

Its focus is on the systematic analysis of naturally occurring talk, whether this talk takes place in informal conversation or formally as conducted in institutional settings. Sidnell and Stivers (2013, p. 2) have identified five distinctive features of conversation analysis:

- It assumes that language use and social interaction more generally are orderly at a minute level of detail; this orderliness is in turn accomplished through methods of reasoning and action shared by the actors.
- The goal of conversation analysis is to describe the overall structure of interactions.
- The data used in analysis are records of spontaneous, naturally occurring interactions, normally audio or video recordings.
- These records (or segments of them) are transcribed in minute detail using a system based on Jeffersonian transcription conventions. The analysis proceeds by focusing on both the original recording and the corresponding transcription. Whereas the recording plays in real time, the transcription allows the analyst to 'freeze' the action in order to 'see' how interaction is organised.
- The analysis itself can be characterised as a qualitative, inductive method. It proceeds as a case-by-case analysis concluding with a series of observations about how normatively social interaction is organised as a collaborative accomplishment by the actors themselves.

At a basic level, there are three principles which underpin the analysis of such naturalistic data and thereby social interaction in general. These principles are:

1. 'if I want to make a contribution to this interaction, then I've got to get a speaking turn';
2. 'once I've got a turn I've got to do something with it';
3. 'I then need to check that the other person understands me and if not correct them'.

These three basic principles correspond to three areas of empirical work unique to conversation analysis: rules of turn taking, sequence organisation of actions in talk and repair.

Turn Taking

As Hayashi notes: 'Turns-at-talk embody opportunities to participate in social life, and as such, are valued and sought after' (Hayashi, 2013, p. 167). Turn taking was an early concern of conversation analysis (Sacks, Schegloff, & Jefferson, 1974), being regarded as a primordial requirement for sociality and the smooth functioning of social interaction and the institutions in which the interaction is played out. This early work identified that there was a system of conventions to which participants oriented, regulating the exchange of turns and management of speaker roles. This system is based the idea of the *Turn Construction Unit* (TCU) which participants understand as a self-contained completed stretch of talk. A TCU can be very short (one word, e.g. 'Fine') or a much longer stretch of talk. Recipients monitor the speaker's talk for the likely end point of a TCU. At these points, there are opportunities for the role of speakership to change to a new speaker or for the current speaker to continue. These opportunity points are known as *Transition Relevance Places* (TRPs). The following is an example of talk from a multidisciplinary meeting where there is a smooth exchange of speakership.

Extract 1: Multidisciplinary Team Meeting: Moving on

(San: Sandra, Meeting chair, Car: Caroline, MDT member)

```
1    San      >Are you happy with the< accuracy::↑=

2    Car      =Yep. Fine.

3    San      (1)>Any further amendment:s (.) ↑then

4             (2)<apart from Jon Taylor:s↑

5             (3)Good

6             (4)Oka:y↓

7             (5)°let's move on°
```

In this segment of talk, we can see how Sandra at line 1 asks a question. This question is delivered as one TCU and in fact selects Caroline as the next speaker since she has earlier suggested an amendment to the minutes of the previous meeting. Caroline is monitoring Sandra's talk and responds seamlessly at the TRP (denoted by the '=' signs at the end and start of each turn) to the question with an affirmation (line 2). Caroline's turn is composed of two TCUs: an immediate affirmation and then a second upgraded evaluation referring to the accuracy of the meeting minutes. These two TCUs are delivered as single words. The completion of Caroline's second TCU creates a TRP which allows Sandra to retake the floor. Sandra's next turn (lines 3–7) is composed of five TCUs (as numbered in the extract). At the end of each where there is a TRP, Sandra self-selects to keep the floor. In sequencing these TCUs in this way, she closes one agenda item and moves on to the next. (See Chapter 4 for a further discussion of this extract.)

In itself, this segment of talk is largely unremarkable; it displays the participants' competence in managing turn taking within the interaction and constituting the encounter as an institutionally based meeting through the coordination of turns and the actions formed in each TCU. However, there are two points to make when considering meeting talk at this level of detail. First, actions performed in each TCU (or combination of TCUs) reflexively constitute the speaker's role within the interaction. The fact that Sandra performs the checking of the minutes, that the other team members recognise this as Sandra's legitimate right as the chair, and that Sandra proposes 'moving on' using an imperative voice (line 6), indicates that the talk itself is a resource for both the participants and the analyst to understand the organisation and accomplishment of these types of meetings. Each turn of talk does three things: it displays the current speaker's understanding of the prior talk; it initiates an action and then sets up a context for a next positioned action.

Second, though this exemplar is potentially mundane and recognisable as a normal sequence of talk in meetings, armed with this understanding, the analyst can identify variations or anomalies to this pattern. For example, as we have noted above, Bokhour (2006) identified meeting practices (giving report, writing report) which seemed to preclude the opportunity for team members to make a contribution of patient information to the formulation of a care plan. A close analysis of turn taking practices of these meetings may well help us understand in more detail how these practices work to limit participation and suggest ways to mitigate them.

Sequence Organisation

One of the fundamental principles of conversation analysis is that talk is action oriented. Talk is not thoughts and ideas simply put into words (Potter & te Molder, 2005), but carefully constructed turns designed to initiate or bring off some actions, such as requesting or giving information, justifying, inviting and so on. These actions have a normative organisation. One of the principal insights of conversation analysis is that these actions are often distributed across two or more people. A basic sequential organisation of talk is in terms of *adjacency pairs*. Adjacency pairs are composed of two turns by different speakers; they are placed one after the other (adjacently); they are relatively ordered; there is first pair part and a second pair part, such that the first initiates a sequence and the second is responsive to the first; and they are also pair typed such that the second is normatively related to the first (e.g. question–answer, invitation–acceptance).

An example of a basic adjacency pair is evident in lines 1–2 of Extract 1. The first pair part is a yes-no-formatted interrogative which sets up the relevance of a second pair part affirming or disconfirming the information requested. A further example which also demonstrates the interaction between turn taking conventions and sequence organisation is shown in the following extract.

Extract 2: Weight Clinic
(Pat: Healthcare professional, Jan: Service user)

```
1   Pat      °let me have a look (1.8) when you were la:ss°

2            (1.8)

3            are ↑you ↑concerned about that ↑weight

4            ↑gain<coz I'm [not]

5   Jan                   [ye:ah]

6            I think it's ↑a [l:ot]

7   Pat                      [ok ] ok

8   Jan:     ↓yeah
```

In line 3, we see Patricia ask a yes-no-formatted interrogative. This first pair part sets up the relevancy of a second pair part agreeing or disagreeing with the inquiry. In line 5, Janis provides the second pair part which is agreement that she is concerned. This is a basic adjacency pair, and in examining the format and content of adjacency pairs, we can get a sense of the agenda and concerns of the organisation members. An additional feature of this interaction which displays how participants both orient to and use as resources turn taking conventions occurs in line 4. The TCU initiating the adjacency pair is: Are you concerned about that weight gain? Completing this TCU creates a TRP where Janis can legitimately provide the second pair part. There is clearly a short delay before Janis starts her TCU. However, before Janis can start, Patricia has very quickly initiated a second TCU. The speed of this start-up is indicated in the transcript by the left carat ('<') indicating that Patricia has pushed the start of her next TCU right up to the end of her first TCU leaving no discernible gap at the TRP. Patricia has claimed the floor at this TRP when normatively the second person would expect to be allocated the floor. Consequently, Janis starts her TCU in overlap with the end of Patricia's second TCU.

Why does this matter?

This short sequence displays the overall ideology of weight management promoted by these healthcare professionals. Through her question design, Patricia has set up confirmation as the preferred second response (see below). She therefore displays that she anticipates this confirmation and quickly steps in to provide her own candidate answer to the question. We can see that Patricia's 'answer' is the direct opposite of Janis'. The healthcare professional in this case is promoting an ideology of 'optimisation' (Heritage, 2010) that is: 'This principle embodies the notion that, unless there is some specific reason not to do so, medical questioning should be designed to allow patients to confirm optimistically framed beliefs and expectation about themselves and their circumstances' (Heritage, 2010, p. 52). Before Janis can provide her own 'pessimistic' response to Patricia's question, Patricia has come in with her own optimistic assessment of Janis' weight gain.

Much work has been conducted on sequence organisation (for a comprehensive summary, see Schegloff, 2007), but two additional points can be made. First, the standard adjacency pair occurs frequently in interaction, but just as frequently we see an expansion of this two-part sequence. There are three ways in which a basic adjacency pair can be expanded: pre-expansion, insert expansion and post-expansion. These forms of expansion provide participants with resources to qualify, resist or develop a line of talk which has been initiated in the interaction.

We saw above how Arber (2008) had examined multidisciplinary team meetings in a palliative care setting. One practice that she noticed was the disproportionate number of questions that nurses asked during the meeting. Here's an example:

Extract 3: Palliative Care Team Meetings (Arber, 2008, p. 1326)

```
1   HPC      Well I just wondered Andrea

2            whether it would be worth trying her

3            on MST 10 milligrams bd?
```

In this case, we see a pre-expansion (line 1) before the first pair part of the adjacency pair (line 2). The conversation analytic literature (Schegloff, 2007) shows us that pre-expansions such as 'Well I just wondered' orient to the delicacy of the substantive matter in hand. This observation allows Arber to conclude that this type of question asking allows nurses to propose treatment courses of action from a position lower in the medical hierarchy compared to doctors.

Finally, going back to Extract 2, we see a post-expansion (line 4). Janis has responded to Patricia's interrogative confirming her concern. She then expands upon this confirmation by explaining that she sees the weight increase as 'a lot'. This expansion seems in part designed to resist the optimising orientation of the healthcare professional and provide an alternative reading of the weight figures that are the focus of the session. If healthcare professionals pursue an optimising ideology, though potentially well-meaning, it runs the risk that service users' own concerns about the treatment or care that they receive are not fully voiced.

A second point is that the types of responses which can be provided as the second pair part are often not equivalent. One type of response can affiliate with the action in the first pair part, whereas another can disaffiliate. An often used example is one of invitation. Acceptance of an invitation affiliates with the action whereas declining the invitation disaffiliates. These two types of response are marked differently in talk. Where the second pair part affiliates with the action, then the response is usually delivered straightforwardly and without delay; this is called a *preferred turn shape*. Conversely where the second pair part disaffiliates with the action, then the response is often delivered with a delay, started with discourse markers (e.g. well), with palliatives and initial appreciations, and accounts; this is called a *dispreferred turn shape* (Pomerantz & Heritage, 2013). In Extract 2, we see the first pair part (line 2) where an affiliative response would be agreement with the assumptions contained in the question, and Janis (in line 3) duly provides a preferred second pair part. Patricia's intervention, before Janis can provide her response, is due to her understanding that a preferred response will be agreement which in turn goes against the optimising ideology that she is pursuing at that point.

Repair

Repair is a participant's mechanism in talk to ensure that an intersubjective understanding of the topic of talk is maintained. Repair is often characterised by a suspension of the smooth progress of talk where one of the participants attends to possible trouble in speaking, hearing or understanding. Conversation analysts have identified two main types of repair: self-initiated repair and other-initiated repair. Self-repair is where the current speaker attends to trouble in their own talk; other-initiated repair is where someone other than the current speaker highlights some trouble and either lets the current speaker use the opportunity to repair their talk or will provide the repair themselves. Overwhelmingly, there is a preference in talk for self-repair (Kitzinger, 2013). The following are two examples of self-repair, both are taken from multidisciplinary team meetings.

Extract 4: Multidisciplinary Team Meeting (1)

Car: Caroline, Meeting chair, San: Sandra, MDT member

```
1  Car      o::ky then harassment how's that done

2  San      it was one of ou:r

3           (.) yea it was still one of our three lowest
```

Extract 5: Multidisciplinary Team Meeting (Bokhour, 2006, p. 358)

```
1   NP     When ac-when you interact with him he's

2          not um, he's not that

3          [{(                    )]

4   OT     [he's not withdrawn]

5   NP     yeah

6   N      He he cries during ADL ADLs in the morning

7          and a lot of times um, you you can talk

8          to him in that and all of a sudden

9          he'll start crying when you're talking

10         to him

11  MD2    There is a [space for    improvement]

12  NP                [His mood is very labile]

13  N      yes

14  MD     that kind of

15         that kind of affect isn't necessarily

16         an indication of depression

17  N      uh huh
```

```
18  MD      You can have inappropr-

19          you can have crying and laughing episodes

20          with these patients with neurologic

21          diseases (in) the so-called frontal sign
```

In Extract 4, the team are discussing some feedback data on their performance and in this segment are focusing on a measure of perceived harassment. In lines 2–3, Sandra self-repairs within the same TCU 'it was one of our' to 'it was still one of our'. She has inserted 'still' into the original phrase. This insertion has the effect of emphasising her understanding and hence this understanding for the other co-present members that this result is a good news story. She emphasises the collegiality of the team (through the use of 'our'—it is a collective achievement) and the continued positive evaluation that can be attributed to the team (through the insertion of 'still').

In Extract 5, the members of a team specialising in the care of patients with Alzheimer's disease are discussing a patient. The nurses and occupational therapist are providing a collaborative first-hand account of this patient's behaviour (lines 1–10). The MD (medical doctor) at line 11 then comes in with a psychiatric explanation of the symptoms. At first, he appears to correct an inference that the first-hand accounts might be leading to a conclusion that the patient is showing symptoms of depression. This response by the MD could be classed as an instance of other repair. This repair gets the go-ahead from one of the nurses (lines 13, 17) which facilitates the MD to elaborate this diagnosis. The MD then self-repairs (lines 18–19). The MD seems set to say 'inappropriate' possibly affect or behaviours, but cuts off and substitutes a different formulation 'you can have crying and laughing episodes...'. The term 'inappropriate' is possibly a demeaning way to label the patient's behaviour, or it is a term which reflects poorly on the care staff who allow such behaviour. In this repair, the MD substitutes an evaluative term for one which is more neutral. As in the previous example, this self-repair may be designed to maintain the collegiality of the team.

Discursive Psychology

Discursive psychology is often viewed as a close intellectual cousin of conversation analysis. A recent definition of discursive psychology is:

> Discursive psychology is a theoretical and analytical approach to discourse which treats talk and text as an object of study in itself, and **psychological concepts as socially managed and consequential in interaction.** (Wiggins, 2017, p. 4. Our emphasis)

The first part of this definition aligns closely with the concerns and interests of conversation analysis. It is the second part of this definition which is a radical development of the conversation analytic project. Discursive psychology assigns a unique status to 'psychological concepts' in so far as they occur in the to and fro of social interaction. Traditionally, psychology has treated psychological terms, such as attitude, belief, emotion and a range of mental processes (memory, attention and so on) as indexing an interior, usually cognitive, process occurring within the mind of the person. In contrast, discursive psychology treats these terms as part of our everyday vocabulary which allow us to pursue certain projects; that is, they can be used to construct versions of events which are action oriented. Discursive psychology focuses on the interactional role and the 'rhetorical affordances' (Edwards, 1997) that such a psychological vocabulary has.

One exemplar of how discursive psychology may be relevant to interprofessional care is to consider the term 'trust'. Trust is a canonical psychological term and one which is conventionally taken to refer to a state of mind existing within a person which influences how they behave towards another in whom they trust. Having 'trust' in someone else would imply that the person would behave towards the other in a cooperative and sympathetic way, giving them licence to behave in ways which might otherwise elicit suspicion in that we would discount them having ulterior motives. By undertaking a brief conceptual analysis of 'trust', we can begin to see the interactional relevance of this concept.

Trust has been invoked by a number of researchers as a precondition for efficient interprofessional collaboration (D'Amour et al., 2005, 2008). These researchers regard trust as a state of mind that can be developed through contact and training with other members allocated to their team. However, a discursive psychology approach would be to examine the use of that term in its discursive context and what its action orientation is. An example of just such discourse comes from D'Amour et al. (2008) study. In developing their model of the organisational and psychological dimensions of collaboration, they identify trust as a state of mind that has to be internalised by the team members. In illustrating the development of trust, they cite members of two teams as follows:

1. 'It's not necessarily that they don't place any trust in the CLSC [Community Health Centre], but if you don't know what goes on in a CLSC, or you know virtually nothing, it's like putting your child into the care of someone you've never met.... If the child is yellow, will they be able to see it's yellow? Will they be able to do their work? It's a demanding approach because neither sector knows the other' (p. 7).
2. 'There was a problem of trust. Even the hospital nurses and the CLSC nurses didn't trust in each other. They questioned each other's competence in caring for the mother or baby. We realize now that the establishments know each other better.... It's still far from perfect, but in terms of harmonizing perinatal care, say, it's a lot better than it was' (p. 8).

If we examine these extracts from a discursive psychology perspective, then our first observation is that they are produced in a research interview. Such talk is then a version of events produced specifically to account for a state of affairs highlighted by the researcher. We can surmise that such versions are designed to display an understanding and rational diagnosis of problems as foregrounded by the researcher. Examining specifically these extracts, we can note in the first that the reference to trust is being used as a disclaimer before the speaker launches into a set of serious criticisms of the current team set-up. Disclaimers are conventionally used to soften the extent of a problematic or sensitive account of events. In the second extract, the term trust is being used as one half of a contrast structure. The 'problem of trust' and the lack of trust in each other is used to construct an extreme, negative version of how events used to be. This version then stands in contrast to the current situation which is 'a lot better than it was'. To conclude, a discursive psychology approach does not treat terms such as trust as pointing unproblematically to a state of mind of the actors, but treats such terms as having rhetorical affordances which enable the speaker to construct versions of events which in turn are action oriented. Moreover, in constructing such versions, the speakers are attentive to how that version reflects upon their own accountability.

Conclusion: Implications for Interprofessional Teamworking

In this chapter, we have outlined the basis for our particular approach to examining multidisciplinary team meetings as the canonical way in which interprofessional care is implemented. Through describing, albeit briefly, conversation analysis and discursive psychology as complementary ways of understanding the dynamics of team meetings, and working through a small number of examples of transcribed interaction, we hope to have demonstrated the analytic utility of these approaches. Practitioners and others new to these ways of analysing talk and text may be surprised by the level of detail on which the analysis focuses. However, it is by noticing and then picking out the moment-to-moment detail of particular instances of interaction and then subjecting them to analysis on a case-by-case basis, that the analyst is able to build a picture of how the participants themselves locally manage their interprofessional work.

This approach to analysis also has very powerful practical and clinical applications. It is becoming increasingly common in the community of conversation analytic practitioners to engage their research participants directly in discussions about the findings. Analysis can be used for training and raising awareness of how the participants manage problematic aspects of their work. A particular approach, CARM (Conversation Analytic Role-play Method, Stokoe, 2011), has been developed for this purpose. It entails identifying instances of interaction which the participants have found problematic in the course of their work and then replaying an instance alongside the transcript. The facilitator breaks the interaction into segments and discusses each step of the interaction with the participants. This approach enables a joint discussion to occur in which the participants both gain a greater understanding of how the details of their talk influence the trajectory of an interaction and also develop ways of dealing with the problematic situation in a different way.

In a variation of this applied approach, some of the authors of the chapters here have engaged their participants at an even earlier stage. They have invited their participants to be involved in 'joint analysis' sessions (see Chapter 14). Such sessions are both enlightening for the participants in so far as they can develop an understanding of the machinery of talk and how that machinery works, as well as informative for the analysts in developing a valid and plausible interpretation of the data.

One caveat to this very direct form of application is that following through on any recommendations for changes in practice will require a degree of organisational diplomacy and negotiation (e.g. Toerien, Irvine, Drew, & Sainsbury, 2011) in order to implement it. Further, we acknowledge that in this book we have examined meetings as the dominant manifestation of interprofessional care; consequently, we pay less attention to other mediums through which interprofessional care can be implemented. In particular, we have not examined more distributed and mediated ways in which it might be implemented, through, for example, electronic communications. Nevertheless, we hope that in this chapter and the others in this book, readers will be able to discern the immense power and value of a detailed analysis of talk in all its manifestations.

References

Arber, A. (2008). Team meetings in specialist palliative care: Asking questions as a strategy within interprofessional interaction. *Qualitative Health Research, 18*(10), 1323–1335. https://doi.org/10.1177/1049732308322588.

Barnard, R. A., Cruice, M. N., & Playford, E. D. (2010). Strategies used in the pursuit of achievability during goal setting in rehabilitation. *Qualitative Health Research, 20*(2), 239–250. https://doi.org/10.1177/1049732309358327.

Bélanger, E., Rodriguez, C., Groleau, D., Légaré, F., Macdonald, M. E., & Marchand, R. (2014). Initiating decision-making conversations in palliative care: An ethnographic discourse analysis. *BMC Palliative Care, 13*: 63. http://www.biomedcentral.com/1472-684X/13/63.

Bokhour, B. G. (2006). Communication in interdisciplinary team meetings: What are we talking about? *Journal of Interprofessional Care, 20*(4), 349–363. https://doi.org/10.1080/13561820600727205.

Brown, B., Crawford, P., & Darongkamas, J. (2000). Blurred roles and permeable boundaries: The experience of multidisciplinary working in community mental health. *Health and Social Care in the Community, 8*(6), 425–435.

Crown Copyright. (2012). *Health and social care act.* London: The Stationary Office.

D'Amour, D., Ferrada-Videla, M., San Martin Rodriguez, L., & Beaulieu, M.-D. (2005). The conceptual basis for interprofessional collaboration: Core concepts and theoretical frameworks. *Journal of Interprofessional Care, 19*(Sup1), 116–131. https://doi.org/10.1080/13561820500082529.

D'Amour, D., Goulet, L., Labadie, J.-F., San Martín-Rodriguez, L., & Pineault, R. (2008). A model and typology of collaboration between professionals in healthcare organizations. *BMC Health Services Research, 2008*(8), 188. https://doi.org/10.1186/1472-6963-8-188.

Deady, R. (2012). Studying multidisciplinary teams in the Irish Republic: The conceptual wrangle. *Perspectives in Psychiatric Care, 48,* 176–182. https://doi.org/10.1111/j.1744-6163.2011.00326.x.

Drew, P., Chatwin, J., & Collins, S. (2001). Conversation analysis: A method for research into interactions between patients and health-care professionals. *Health Expectations, 4,* 58–70.

Edwards, D. (1997). *Discourse and cognition.* London: Sage.

Edwards, D., & Potter, J. (1992). *Discursive psychology.* London: Sage.

Edwards, D., & Potter, J. (2005). Discursive psychology, mental states and descriptions. In H. te Molder & J. Potter (Eds.), *Conversation and cognition*. Cambridge: Cambridge University Press.

Field, K. M., Rosenthal, M. A., Dimou, J., Fleet, M., Gibbs, P., & Drummond, K. (2010). Communication in and clinician satisfaction with multidisciplinary team meetings in neuro-oncology. *Journal of Clinical Neuroscience, 17*, 1130–1135.

Finn, R., Learmonth, M., & Reedy, P. (2010). Some unintended effects of teamwork in healthcare. *Social Science and Medicine, 70*, 1148–1154. https://doi.org/10.1016/j.socscimed.2009.12.025.

Hayashi, M. (2013). Turn allocation and turn sharing. In J. Sidnell & T. Stivers (Eds.), *Handbook of conversation analysis*. Chichester: Wiley-Blackwell.

Hepburn, H., & Bolden, G. (2013). The conversation analytic approach to transcription. In J. Sidnell & T. Stivers (Eds.), *Handbook of conversation analysis*. Chichester: Wiley-Blackwell.

Heritage, J. (2010). Questioning in medicine. In A. F. Freed & S. Ehrlich (Eds.), *"Why do you ask?": The function of questions in institutional discourse*. Oxford: Oxford University Press.

Heritage, J., Robinson, J. D., Elliot, M., Beckett, M., & Wilkes, M. (2007). Reducing patients' unmet concerns: The difference one word can make. *Journal of General Internal Medicine, 22*, 1429–1433.

Kitzinger, C. (2013). Repair. In J. Sidnell & T. Stivers (Eds.), *Handbook of conversation analysis*. Chichester: Wiley-Blackwell.

Kuziemsky, C. E., Borycki, E. M., Purkis, M. E., Black, F., Boyle, M., ..., Interprofessional Practices Team. (2009). An interdisciplinary team communication framework and its application to healthcare 'e-teams' systems design. *BMC Medical Informatics and Decision Making, 9*, 43. https://doi.org/10.1186/1472-6947-9-43.

Lewin, S., & Reeves, S. (2011). Enacting 'team' and 'teamwork': Using Goffman's theory of impression management to illuminate interprofessional practice on hospital wards. *Social Science and Medicine, 72*, 1595–1602. https://doi.org/10.1016/j.socscimed.2011.03.037.

O'Carroll, V., McSwiggan, L., & Campbell, M. (2016). Health and social care professionals' attitudes to interprofessional working and interprofessional education: A literature review. *Journal of Interprofessional Care, 30*(1), 42–49. https://doi.org/10.3109/13561820.2015.1051614.

Pillay, B., Wootten, A. C., Crowe, H., Corcoran, N., Tran, B., Bowden, P., ... & Costello, A. J. (2016). The impact of multidisciplinary team meetings on patient assessment, management and outcomes in oncology settings: A systematic review of the literature. *Cancer Treatment Reviews, 42*, 56–72.

Pomerantz, A., & Heritage, J. (2013). Preference. In J. Sidnell & T. Stivers (Eds.), *Handbook of conversation analysis*. Chichester: Wiley-Blackwell.

Potter, J., & Hepburn, A. (2005). Qualitative interviews in psychology: Problems and possibilities. *Qualitative Research in Psychology, 2*, 281–307.

Potter, J., & Hepburn, A. (2012). Eight challenges for interview researchers. In J. F. Gubrium, J. A. Holstein, A. B. Marvasti, & K. D. McKinney (Eds.), *The Sage handbook of interview research: The complexity of the craft* (2nd ed.). Thousand Oaks, CA: Sage.

Potter, J., & te Molder, H. (2005). Talking cognition: Making and mapping the terrain. In H. te Molder & J. Potter (Eds.), *Conversation and cognition*. Cambridge: Cambridge University Press.

Reeves, S., Lewin, S., Espin, S., & Zwarenstein, M. (2010). *Interprofessional teamwork for health and social care*. Chichester: Wiley-Blackwell.

Reeves, S., Xyrichis, A., & Zwarenstein, M. (2018). Teamwork, collaboration, coordination, and networking: Why we need to distinguish between different types of interprofessional practice. *Journal of Interprofessional Care, 32*(1), 1–3. https://doi.org/10.1080/13561820.2017.1400150.

Rice, K., Zwarenstein, M., Conn, L. G., Kenaszchuk, C., Russell, A., & Reeves, S. (2010). An intervention to improve interprofessional collaboration and communications: A comparative qualitative study. *Journal of Interprofessional Care, 24*, 350–361. https://doi.org/10.3109/13561820903550713.

Roulston, K. (2011). Working through challenges in doing interview research. *International Journal of Qualitative Methods, 10*(4), 348–366.

Sacks, H. (1992). *Lectures on conversation* (2 vols.). Oxford: Basil Blackwell.

Sacks, H., Schegloff, E., & Jefferson, G. (1974). A simplest systematics for the organization of turn taking for conversation. *Language, 50*, 696–735.

Schegloff, E. (2007). *Sequence organization in interaction: A primer in conversation analysis*. Cambridge: Cambridge University Press.

Sidnell, J. (2010). *Conversation analysis: An introduction*. Chichester: Wiley-Blackwell.

Sidnell, J., & Stivers, T. (Eds.). (2013). *Handbook of conversation analysis*. Chichester: Wiley-Blackwell.

Stokoe, E. (2011). Simulated interaction and communication skills training: The 'Conversation-Analytic Role-Play Method'. In C. Antaki (Ed.), *Applied conversation analysis: Intervention and change in institutional talk*. London: Palgrave Macmillan.

The Mid Staffordshire NHS Foundation Trust Public Inquiry. (2013). *Report of the Mid Staffordshire NHS Foundation Trust Public Inquiry: Executive summary* (Chaired by Robert Francis QC). London: The Stationery Office.

Toefien, M., Irvine, A., Drew, P., & Sainsbury, R. (2011). Should mandatory jobseeker interviews be personalised? The politics of using conversation analysis to make effective practice recommendations. In C. Antaki (Ed.), *Applied conversation analysis: Intervention and change in institutional talk*. London: Palgrave Macmillan.

Watson, C., & Drew, V. (2017). Humour and laughter in meetings: Influence, decision-making and the emergence of leadership. *Discourse and Communication, 11*(3), 314–329. https://doi.org/10.1177/1750481317699432.

Wiggins, S. (2017). *Discursive psychology: Theory, method and applications*. London: Sage.

Wittenberg-Lyles, E., Oliver, D. P., Demiris, G., & Regehr, K. (2010). Interdisciplinary collaboration in hospice team meetings. *Journal of Interprofessional Care, 24*(3), 264–273. https://doi.org/10.3109/13561820903163421.

Zwarenstein, M., Goldman J., & Reeves, S. (2009). Interprofessional collaboration: Effects of practice-based interventions on professional practice and healthcare outcomes. *Cochrane Database of Systematic Reviews* (3). Art. No.: CD000072. https://doi.org/10.1002/14651858.cd000072.pub2.

3

Healthcare Meetings Where the Service User Is Absent: The Ethical and Values-Based Implications for Research

Cordet Smart, Lindsay Aikman, Madeleine Tremblett, Jennifer Dickenson and Sifiso Mhlanga

Introduction

but I thought Conversation Analysis was a cold method that seems to remove the emotion and experience from an interaction

This was the opinion of conversation analysis expressed to me (CS) by a clinical psychologist prior to a one-hour workshop. The topic of the workshop was to discuss why conversation analysis (CA) was useful for understanding team meetings and formulation. I recall a sense of trepidation at this very early presentation in the life of the *MDTsInAction* research programme, but once I put up some of my data on the PowerPoint and gave the participants the written transcript, they quickly engaged. The challenges seemed to centre on the ethics of

C. Smart (✉) · M. Tremblett
School of Psychology, University of Plymouth, Plymouth, UK
e-mail: cordet.smart@plymouth.ac.uk

M. Tremblett
e-mail: madeleine.tremblett@plymouth.ac.uk

© The Author(s) 2018
C. Smart and T. Auburn (eds.), *Interprofessional Care and Mental Health*,
The Language of Mental Health, https://doi.org/10.1007/978-3-319-98228-1_3

undertaking a forensic examination of interaction, seemingly stripping away emotion and how this could be considered as ethical or values-based practice: how could this be compassionate? Further, was it really ethical to study contexts about service users, where they were not present? The authenticity of exploring and understanding *real-life* interactions, however, seemed to be what they ultimately valued.

Studying an MDT meeting raised so many discussion points. There was the potential for those involved as participants to feel exposed, handing over recordings of their behaviours with nothing to hide behind and having to tolerate the uncertainty of what might be made of it. It was crucial to be sensitive in the management of data, application and dissemination of findings. By strong values base and highest ethical standards, we do not simply mean working within an ethically approved project framework but rather, how to approach all components of the research: processes of consultation with service users, carers and staff participants; ways of talking about the project (being accurate and reassuring around an unfamiliar methodology); sensitivity to power imbalances in recruitment; selection of focal interactional patterns; and methods of feeding back.

This chapter follows the book format of providing an introduction, in which we will elaborate the main contexts that seemed to influence ethical dilemmas and then a project overview. It offers a generic overview of the project from the perspective of the ethical protocol. The 'findings' presented here are reflections from different researchers around some of the key areas of implementation. The chapter aims to offer an accessible understanding of how to consider

L. Aikman
Livewell Southwest, Plymouth, UK
e-mail: lindsay.aikman@nhs.net

J. Dickenson
Devon Partnership NHS Trust, Exeter, UK
e-mail: jenniferdickenson@nhs.net

S. Mhlanga
Leicestershire Partnership Trust, Leicester, UK
e-mail: sifiso.mhlanga@nhs.net

and manage some of the ethical concerns that might be encountered in conducting research like this, and to contribute to the newly developing literature around managing the ethics of qualitative research in mental health care.

Main Ethical Issues

We identified three main contexts as having a significant impact in our consideration of ethical issues.

Wider Ethical Issues in (Qualitative) Mental Healthcare Research

This section considers dilemmas arising from benchmarking qualitative research against its quantitative counterparts, the impact of developments in service user involvement, issues of confidentiality and the consequences of researching clinical contexts.

Cohen and Crabtree (2008) highlight that one of the main challenges of qualitative research when trying to establish any benchmarks for quality has been its extremely diverse nature. Qualitative research has been applied with increasing rigour in health care globally (Salmon, 2013), and this has meant that ethics boards are continuously presented with new ethical dilemmas. Many of these dilemmas do not fit with the standardised protocols that have historically been appropriate for clinical trials (Cohen & Crabtree, 2008; Pollock, 2012; Sanjari, Bahramnezhad, Fomani, Shoghi, & Cheraghi, 2014; Stevenson, Gibson, Pelletier, Chrysikou, & Park, 2015). It seems essential, therefore, that these issues are continuously reflected on and re-addressed. Stevenson et al. (2015) propose that the main ethical issue is that qualitative research often focuses on process rather than outcomes. The current benchmark assessments therefore generally judge qualitative research as poor, because qualitative research is designed to explore relationships, rather than identifying definitive outcomes. This difference in understanding of qualitative research in ethics processes also means that some areas of ethical concern receive less sophisticated consideration. For example, Sanjari et al. (2014) highlight several issues, including the different ethical issues that arise from the interpretation of the data by researchers and subsequently by consumers of the research. In some ways, discursive psychology (DP) has sought specifically to be rigorous, to develop a careful corpus of normative data and highlight normative practices, which ensures that findings always have a baseline in established social practices. Yet, this needs to be tempered by a values-based awareness of how service users might receive these findings.

We suggest that public and patient involvement (PPI) is one of the most significant areas of ethical consideration for qualitative (and all) research in mental health contexts. In the UK in 2001, it became a legal requirement for service users to be consulted in research and the development of all health services, yet the implementation of this requirement seems to have been slow (Crane, 2018). Within clinical research, there has been a slow transition as a consequence, from research on people, to with, and currently increasingly done 'by' people, as Milner and Frawley (2018) discuss for people with learning disabilities. However, there is limited robust research exploring the impact of PPI on healthcare and social care research (Brett et al., 2014). There are a number of ways that multiple stakeholders, that is commissioners, service users, carers, clinicians and beyond, might be involved in research. Brett et al. (2014) reviewed 68 papers which they grouped into four areas. They suggest that stakeholders might be part of the initial consultation, design of questionnaires, act as co-analysts or people who might check the quality of findings and partake in writing, reviewing and dissemination. In particular, they found that there was potential for significant enhancement of the quality and relevance of the research. NHS (National Health Service) ethics in the UK also requires an element of consultation for all applications, with queries raised if this has not been done. There are broader debates around different forms of engagement—consultation before research is done, as a steering group during the research process and as an evaluation group of the research. Stakeholders can also be involved in data collection or data analysis. In qualitative research, we are able to involve people perhaps more at this final level. However, some key challenges include how the quality of analysis is maintained, managing the involvement so that it is presented in a balanced way, and cost implications (Brett et al., 2014).

The emphasis on PPI gives rise to a context not just of service users being involved in research, but also for research that focuses directly on contexts that involve service users. This presented a challenge for *MDTsInAction*. We felt that *not* studying interactions where service users are absent would lead to an oversight, however, and perhaps even a false representation of the way the usual practice within health services is conducted.

Confidentiality and data protection became a further major issue for our research. With quantitative data, it is more feasible to anonymise data pertaining to people. With qualitative work such as ours, voices of research participants are identifiable; further, we were observing people's everyday practices. This issue was particularly sensitive at the time of this research (2014–2018); as following the Berwick/Francis reports of 2014, the NHS in the UK seems to have entered a culture of blame. There are constant conversations around the quality of practice, which is always under scrutiny, and thus, the emphasis on confidentiality was heightened, with a real concern about 'revealing' information and practices.

It was also important here to consider who was conducting the research. Relating to the clinical context can be one of the greatest challenges to research in the NHS, which is where we started at the beginning of the chapter. It seemed appropriate to be sensitive to the pressures inherent in mental healthcare settings and take care to not impose an academic understanding on how the research protocol might work. This is particularly the case when we consider the history of mental health care, which, in the UK alone, has taken some considerable journey from placing people in asylums and providing care from a medicalised approach. Current trends provide new understandings through validating personal meanings in mental health care, as illustrated by the recent Power Threat and Meaning Framework published by Johnstone et al. (2018).

Ethical Issues Raised Through a Focus on MDTs Where Service Receivers/Users and Carers Are absent

The second issue that produced ethical concerns was that we sought to study meetings where service users and carers were absent. This directly challenged the ethos of the healthcare context that we were working which emphasised how service users should be involved at all stages of their care. At times during ethical and consultation processes, it has seemed almost shameful to mention that our research programme is about contexts where service users are not present. These 'professional-only meetings' form a regular part of the day-to-day functioning of services where typically multiple service users are discussed, and therefore, it is not commonplace for service users to be invited as individual care was not discussed in detail. Further, to ignore their existence would seem inauthentic when the aim is to study the ways in which health professionals operate as a team.

There is an entire 'backstage' as Lewin and Reeves (2011) term it that may become inaccessible to study because it does not quite fit with the image of healthcare practice that services may wish to portray. However, research examining contexts where the service user voice is only present through the intervention of others suggests the importance of examining the organisation and day-to-day operation of such services. Further reasons to support research of professional-only meetings include challenging the assumption that pressure for service users and their carers to be present at every meeting would be welcome. It is also about recognising the value for clinicians to have opportunities to discuss the quality of care provision and to raise concerns with the team around service user care (see Chapter 4 for further consideration of the function these meetings may serve for staff).

Studying the multidisciplinary context directly enabled a consideration of how different voices are heard. This does fit with current policy drivers emphasising the importance of effective communication and joint working between professionals. Furthermore, it also complements the global interprofessional working and education agendas, as discussed in Chapter 1. However, this raised further issues around consent to participate in the research from the service users who are discussed in meetings, particularly as some service users might have had differing capacities to consent. Long discussions were held within the research team and with stakeholders on this issue. However, consultation with the NHS research ethics committee, along with service users and carers, suggested that this could in fact be unethical, as it would not affect their care directly, and could increase the pressure on service users, potentially leaving them feeling distressed. Equally, in some mental health services, service users may present with difficulties related to trusting professionals, and therefore, it was not judged to be helpful to seek the informed consent of the absent service users.

Qualitative/Discursive Method of Analysis

The methodological framework of qualitative discursive approaches raised its own ethical and values-based dilemmas. The first dilemma emerges around the use of CA, which arguably can create an inherent power imbalance. CA is often considered as a highly skilled form of analysis, which implies that only those with skills to analyse conversations can complete analysis. This conflicts at some level with notions of joint analysis and how service user involvement might be achieved.

Secondly, CA, as discussed in Chapter 2, prioritises naturalistic data. There seems to be an assumption that studying naturalistic data is in some sense more ethical as it is dealing directly with the interaction of the participants. Using extracts as part of the analysis allows the reader more or less direct access to the interaction which forms the basis of the analysis. However, there is an inherent conflict here between being respectful of privacy and the opening up of the details of how people actually talk.

The CA approach also develops that sense of clinicians being watched, and there were occasions when an orientation to the presence of the recording devices was apparent. There also needed to be a careful awareness that the public nature of recording might make any person who had reservations about engaging in the research feel revealed and therefore not fully engage in discussions during the meetings. This is not to say that we did not carefully seek consent from the meeting members individually and fully discuss the implications. However, inevitably, it is likely that some people felt unsure. We therefore had to be very careful to be clear that CA is not of itself evaluative, but seeks to reveal how things work, rather than to judge performance.

Project Overview

Here, we provide an overview of the generic research protocol, from consultation to dissemination, with an ethical focus. For this chapter, our 'findings' are not outputs, but rather reflections from researchers from different stages of the research project. For this research programme, which was conducted within the UK, we engaged in a number of different processes to gain ethical approval. Initially, we took the proposed research idea (gaining a better understanding of interprofessional collaboration between staff in meetings) to a service user group that was attached to the university (see also Chapter 13). There had been a number of discussions around poor communication, and we felt that our research would be a useful response to these.

Formal ethical approvals were gained through a combination of university and NHS bodies, which later became the HRA (UK healthcare ethics governance body). There were a number of discussions as to whether we needed specialist confidentiality governance, as this project involved the direct recording of team meetings, and might include patient data. However, it was agreed that the approach would be acceptable because the study would involve data anonymisation within 72 hours, with short snippets of data as the analytic focus, and an emphasis on staff interactions not service users' problems.

There were also complex discussions around data storage, and eventually, a secure online cloud storage was identified. The logistics of recording, storing and then transferring the data to the cloud were very clearly specified.

We met with teams to discuss the research. If they agreed to take part, then we returned for a second meeting and sought informed consent. Recording devices were left with a named team member. Staff could individually opt out and we would destroy the data; however, we encountered no instances of this.

After the research, we sent summaries of the findings to the teams, and where possible, met to conduct joint analysis and to discuss their experiences of participation. Finally, training sessions were offered to some teams based on the overall findings in an attempt to give something back to staff for their participation. We felt that this training was particularly valuable in a climate of funding cuts. Participants were also asked for contributions to the book.

Researcher Reflections

An Unusual Ethical Proposition?—Lindsay Aikman

At the beginning of the research programme, things were less clear, and the negotiation of ethics approvals was challenging. I recall the constant difficult questions raised. The main dilemma was that the research fell between guidelines. Within the UK at that time, if you recruited *service user* participants from NHS services, it was clear that NHS ethical approval was needed, but if only *staff* were included, then approval from your research institution was sufficient. Our question was what happens when your participants are NHS staff, but by virtue of it being naturalistic data you are potentially exposed to 'patient-identifiable' information? This represents a possible violation of the sanctity of confidentiality, yet this data capturing would be inadvertent and not part of the research itself. It was the answering of this question that underpinned much of the early consultation undertaken, as reflected on below, where I consider the different perspectives of stakeholders.

Ethical considerations for service users and carers. As you will hear from fellow researchers, each project sought out meaningful consultation with service users and carers. In my own case (see Chapter 6), this discussion centred around acceptability of researchers having access to 'patient-identifiable' data in the course of listening to the recorded meetings.

Service users considered this acceptable to them, as identifying data would be removed, was not the focus of the study and that care is discussed in these meetings anyway. They fed back that the research seemed valuable because it promoted joined-up care, and lack of joined-up care is what many of them described as contributing to their unhelpful healthcare experiences. They suggested this research might improve service user experience of NHS services by shining a light on practices that take place behind closed doors. I sensed there was some reference to addressing a general power imbalance service users acknowledged at the prospect of being discussed by professionals without knowing what is said.

Whilst encouraging, we also needed to have our potential exposure to information regarding people's care considered and approved through formal bodies. The next paragraph comes from our formal advice from the NHS ethics committee. Please feel free to read it quickly, but I include it in full to demonstrate the shared lack of clarity around how to hold this ethical dilemma responsibly. The particular ethical processes change over time but in broad terms:

> We sought advice from a body called the Confidentiality Advisory Group (CAG) who advised seeking the more stringent NHS ethics but their proportionate (partial) review rather than a full Research Ethics Committee application. This sub-committee subsequently determined that they were unable to make the decision and that there were 'material ethical issues' requiring the fullest ethical review; this included defending the project at panel. At this next panel, their considered opinion was that the impact of gaining informed from every patient raised in conversation would itself be **unethical** given that we were reviewing NHS staff interactions and any reference to patients as part of these interactions would be anonymised at the earliest opportunity.

Following this letter, full ethical approval was sought, and granted, by the research institution. After 81 emails were exchanged with R&D departments across 5 NHS trusts (now replaced by a single HRA application), my project could begin. This experience, the complexity, confusion and at times frustration that surrounded it, made apparent the lack of certainty about how to responsibly approach projects such as this. Was this really such an unusual ethical proposition?

Ethical considerations for participants—staff. One of the reasons teams were keen to support the research was captured by a comment from one team lead—that the work of MDT teams is constantly under threat because it is an expensive activity and it is hard to explain what it does in concrete terms. I had to hold in mind that teams may have been participating on the basis that they hoped the research would support their arguments in a positive way. This had to be balanced against what the data showed in terms of patterns emerging.

Professionals expressed some vulnerability about having their team conversations explored in detail. There was concern regarding having a 'dark' sense of humour, used by teams to help them cope with the stresses of their work, and that comments might be taken out of context. As researchers, we were able to offer some reassurances in response to these concerns. For example, that our analysis would consider carefully the context, that the research was based on the practices of multiple teams, and that all extracts used in the analysis would be brief and anonymous. However, it was also relevant to reflect on the value that some level of feeling 'exposed' could have, in enabling reflection on how to develop clinical practice. At that stage, it was unclear quite what might fall under the label of 'dark humour' and there was an ethical obligation to act upon content if it was inappropriate. The team accepted this and seemed to appreciate the clear boundaries set.

Teams were conscious of being recorded and I had hoped that the project was set up in a way that allowed people to engage in their meeting practice as normal. I was pleased that two teams took the opportunity to pause recordings during segments that they did not want to have recorded. In both cases, these centred around staffing issues within their team and recruitment-based conversations. Other than this, teams seemed to forget quite quickly that the recording devices were there and went about conducting their meeting unproblematically. I asked every team member to sign a consent form at each meeting to ensure people were willing and informed at multiple points. No one subsequently fed back issues of discomfort or requested to withdraw from the study. Does that automatically mean everyone was fully happy to participate?

Ethical considerations for the researcher. There was a high degree of subjectivity in identifying focal interactional practices once data were collected. I noted my own anxiety at being drawn to how frustration was expressed in meetings and how this might be challenging for team members to later read about—perhaps reflecting some of my own discomfort with conflict more generally and dis-ease reconciling this against my gratitude at their willingness to participate. Through the use of bracketing interviews, a technique commonly used in qualitative interviews to mitigate the damaging impact of researcher bias, I acknowledged that I didn't want to restrict the analysis to only those patterns that felt safe and cautious. It also helped me be thoughtful about remaining focused on clinical implications of interactions and write up the analysis respectfully.

It was from this basis of uncertainty that the research programme developed and evolved to enhance an understanding of how ethics and values worked within it. Jenny illustrates this from a later project.

My Experiences with Seeking Meaningful Service User and Carer Consultation—Jennifer Dickenson

Consultation with service users and carers was incorporated into my research process (see Chapter 10) to gain feedback on the proposed research and try to increase the impact of the research. My experience consisted of approaching a specific service user and carer consultative group linked with a university. This quarterly meeting consisted of different service users, carers, trainee clinical psychologists and staff within the university coming together. In addition to other consultation contributions this group made to the doctorate in clinical psychology, this meeting also provided a forum where researchers could share prospective study ideas and gain consultation and feedback from the service user and carer consultative group.

During the process of consultation, several challenges were identified. DP/CA is revealing of everyday practices, and on occasions critical of social institutions, it can also be restrictive owing to the expert knowledge required by analysts. During my consultation experiences, it is often felt difficult to try and communicate the research aims at a level that was accessible to the audience. This may highlight a barrier when trying to incorporate meaningful consultation for research where CA is the analytic method.

I also became aware that all of the service users had their own experiences of accessing services and were at different stages in their journey. This sometimes resulted in people becoming focused on their own experiences, and therefore, the attention was taken away from specifically discussing the proposed research. I feel my preparation prior to attending the consultation could have been improved if I had prepared more specific questions to better equip me to direct the conversation and stay focused upon the proposed research. If I had spent more time considering how to make the consultation more meaningful, this could have also made better use of the allocated time. It may be helpful to gain feedback from the service users and carers on how they felt that specific consultation went. For example, how clearly the research was explained, if they felt heard and understood? This may then help to shape future consultations. This may also help to draw clarity on what motivates the researcher to gain consultation and help to reduce consultation from feeling or appearing tokenistic.

This experience was helpful in two ways in particular; firstly, it provided a valued space for service users and carers to voice some of their experiences and perspectives of not being present at meetings, and secondly, in doing so, it shaped the focus of the analysis. The analysis in Chapter 10 focuses on how the experiences of the service user and carer are shared during the MDT meetings when they were not physically present or invited. Overall, the consultation appeared to provide a space for service users and carers to talk about their experiences and perspectives of being absent from MDTs.

Gatekeepers and Unintentional Power Effects in Recruitment—Madeleine Tremblett

The recruitment of staff members for our research on multidisciplinary teams in the NHS has led to a number of ethical reflections. I have visited multiple teams to present our research and have engaged in discussions with the teams to see if they would like to take part. In one such meeting, a staff member jokingly asked '*I tend to swear quite a lot in these meetings – you won't feed this back to our boss will you?*' I will use this comment to illustrate some of the ethical issues discussed by the *MDTsInAction* team when staff are participants. First, I will reflect on the role of gatekeepers to the team and subsequently reflect on the staff's involvement in the research process.

Gatekeepers who determine our access to the participants necessary for this research have a considerable and powerful role. The power they hold predominately originates from a manager–subordinate relationship. The gatekeeper of the research strand I was involved with was the head of service for a county. I held meetings with them to demonstrate the value of the research and reassure them of the minimal impact involvement would have on the teams' day-to-day work. Luckily, the head of the service was enthusiastic about the research and agreed that this was something the teams could be involved with. Contact details for the team leaders in their service were provided by this gatekeeper to allow us to arrange meetings with the individual teams. The head of service asked to be copied into emails sent to team leaders, however, to enable them to keep track of the research, and as such, the team leaders would have an awareness of the service manager's endorsement of the research. On reflection, this knowledge may have affected the team leaders' freedom of choice to allow us to present the research to their team. It is of course important that they knew the research had official permission, yet knowledge of the head of service's endorsement may equally have led to a sense of obligation to allow us access to the team. The comment, 'you won't feed this back to our boss will you?', demonstrates awareness of the gatekeeper's involvement and the potential for unintentional power effects.

Although the head of service acts as the main gatekeeper to the teams, the team leaders, in turn, act as gatekeepers to the team members. As soon as the meeting had been arranged, staff members could consider this as endorsement of the research by the team leader as well as the head of service. The team leader may even have mentioned to the staff members that this has been approved by the head of service. The comment presented above suggests this may have been the case for my research. 'Our boss' is referenced in the comment, and as the team leader was present, 'our boss' implies the boss of both the team and team leader. Again, this may lead to a power imbalance where staff members may feel some obligation to take part, as both their manager and the head of service have determined our research to be a worthwhile activity for the team.

These hierarchical structures within an organisation are hard to avoid. We would not be able to do the research in the NHS without getting the approvals from the head of service in the first place. However, as also raised by Flewitt (2005), it is concerning that staff members may feel obliged to consent to take part because they feel it is the right thing to do in their job role, rather than as something they feel comfortable doing. Flewitt (2005) suggests that the way to overcome this is to ensure there are safe, as well as formal and informal, ways that participants are able to decline to take part. For our research, we do get team consent overall to begin with, as well as obtaining informed consent from individuals in one-to-one meetings. Each staff member is also provided with our contact details to withdraw their participation at any time. Yet, in busy teams, the one-to-one meetings are often rushed and lack engagement from team members who are eager to get on with their job roles. As such, the onus is on us as researchers to ensure that the time is protected and that staff do have an opportunity to fully understand what they are consenting to.

A further dilemma in healthcare research is the value given to staff when they are the main participants. For our research, it was necessary for us to get validation of the research aims from a service users and carers group. However, this consultation did not occur with the actual staff members who were our participants. Instead, they only experienced the presentation and information sheets given during recruitment. Although it is important to consult service users and carers, as the hope is that research findings may impact beneficially on the care they receive, staff participants may also add important issues at the research design stage. The current practice of not doing a staff consultation seems to devalue what their potential input could be. Furthermore, as the initial comment made by a staff member suggests, staff may not fully understand the research that we are doing. The comment implies that we might be looking to be critical of individual staff members and their behaviour. However, our research looks at interactional practices that are common across groups; we do not want, nor would it be feasible, to look at specific staff members. Yet, the comment made suggests this message did not come across clearly to the staff in the recruitment presentation. Thus, consulting staff and involving them in research at an earlier stage may help ensure that the information we provide is clear and understandable to someone without a research background.

Ending the Research Relationship with Stakeholders—Cordet Smart and Sifiso Mhlanga

A final reflective point that we wanted to raise was around endings. Quite often in research, we discuss a 'debrief' after the research, but this does not really fit with a qualitative paradigm. Endings are also not often considered but are especially important when effective working relationships had been developed with clinicians with an interest in engaging in future research. The importance of endings for us came mostly from the feeling after collecting the data, transcribing and working on the analysis, that there seemed to be something missing—the voice of the clinicians involved. One of the interesting issues in this research was that, within the zeitgeist of contemporary healthcare contexts, it is very easy to be aware of the service user and to foreground them, surprisingly even when the person was not physically present within the meeting. However, it was easy in this research to overlook the participants—the clinicians themselves as stakeholders and as appropriate consultants within the research.

Consequently, opportunities to ask participants and other managers about their thoughts and experiences of taking part in the research became really valuable. Managers wanted to know what the key single 'points' were that they might be able to apply. Clinicians wanted to know how they could better organise their meetings and communicate with each other particularly within services where clinicians managed a high caseload and needed to use their time effectively. They were keen and enthusiastic to discuss the findings and seemed to enjoy the opportunity to continue to develop their practice. Leaving was still hard—they wanted more analysis meetings, and it would have been beneficial to be able to have run more training sessions. It would be important to plan for future research to include more consultation with clinicians who were participants, ensuring mutually beneficial timing for feedback. Careful consideration was also needed in terms of how to feedback to other stakeholders who were not directly involved in the research, e.g. service managers. We did this using summaries of findings approved by participants.

A central concern was how to present sensitive feedback to teams who had so kindly given consent for us to conduct the research. It is good to discuss this at greater length during the consent process, and as the programme evolved, we became increasingly aware of the importance of being entirely open and honest. It was helpful in later studies to ask teams how they feel about this, and how they want information to be shared. In our experience, the feedback sessions were validating for clinicians and provided discussion opportunities (see Chapters 15 and 16). This validation often seemed a relief, or even in part a surprise for participants. However, at some points, the styles of interacting presented seemed to have unexpected effects. For example, in one meeting the chair had sought to make things more informal, not including an agenda, which seemed to increase the number of 'bids' for leadership of the meeting, interrupting meeting progression. Hearing this seemed to give participants space to reflect on the running of the meeting. Our analysis seemed to reveal different practices that clinicians could then discuss.

For some clinicians, the process of being involved in the feedback brought up anxiety about the implications of the research and how the findings would be applied. There were dilemmas around sharing with senior managers and how to delicately achieve this. This was especially important as the senior managers were often involved at the initial consultation stage and essentially acted as gatekeepers, but were not present themselves during the meetings that were recorded and analysed in this research. Feedback was therefore arranged with groups of clinicians who had taken part in the research to create a 'collective experience'. This enabled discussion of publication intentions, and all feedback was designed to explore generic patterns, not to identify individual poor performance.

Recommendations for Interprofessional Team Working

- Ethical dilemmas in research in interprofessional working should be directly and openly discussed—we need to constantly balance the benefits and challenges of the research.
- Reflection on ethical issues, such as the openness and revealing nature of the research process, was interesting as a way of interrogating practice—for researchers and clinicians.
- Reflecting on the power disparities inherent in research processes might help people to understand their preferences for or against research participation.

Summary

This chapter sought to highlight some of the ethical considerations in conducting a study of staff team functioning in mental health-care contexts. It presented a review of the particular trident of characteristics: the method, mental healthcare ethical context and the topic, having service users were in absentia, that lead to a very particular ethical complex. We think that exploring these issues is crucial for the continued development of the use of discursive research methods within mental health contexts. It appears important for the development of both—in terms of discursive research practice it can make researchers seem more 'human' and to be aware that it is not just 'discourse' that is being studied, but people in complex social worlds, who need sensitive treatment. For healthcare contexts, issues around openness and access to what happens in everyday practice are opened up. Revealing practice can be anxiety provoking, but also lends itself to a different form of reflection which might help to reveal new insights to practices and challenges that individuals are having with practice, through enabling them to stand outside of, and directly observe, their own practice.

Tips for doing research
Use the process of gaining ethical approval and thinking about ethics to consider the meaning of your research
Try not to resist changes suggested by participants because they 'don't understand a research method' or those suggested by a researcher who is not a clinician as they 'don't understand the clinical context'. Use the feedback to think through different, new approaches
Develop simple and accessible ways of explaining your project—both those for more in-depth consultation conversations and an 'elevator pitch' for ad hoc discussions around your research
Draw on the ethical considerations from previous projects to inform your thinking
Sometimes ethics boards might not have come across your techniques—try to use them for advice, and look at other projects and how they have managed ethical concerns

References

Brett, J., Staniszewska, S., Mockford, C., Herron-Marx, S., Hughes, J., Tysall, C., & Suleman, R. (2014). Mapping the impact of patient and public involvement on health and social care research: A systematic review. *Health Expectations, 17*(5), 637–650.

Cohen, D. J., & Crabtree, B. F. (2008). Evaluative criteria for qualitative research in health care: Controversies and recommendations. *The Annals of Family Medicine, 6*(4), 331–339.

Crane, J. (2018). Why the history of public consultation matters for contemporary health policy. *Endeavour, 42*(1), 9–16. https://doi.org/10.1016/j.endeavour.2018.01.001.

Flewitt, R. (2005). Conducting research with young children: Some ethical considerations. *Early Child Development and Care, 175*(6), 553–565.

Johnstone, L., Boyle, M., Cromby, J., Dillon, J., Harper, D., Kinderman, P., …, Read, J. (2018). *The power threat meaning framework: Towards the identification of patterns in emotional distress, unusual experiences and troubled or troubling behaviour, as an alternative to functional psychiatric diagnosis.* Leicester: British Psychological Society.

Lewin, S., & Reeves, S. (2011). Enacting 'team' and 'teamwork': Using Goffman's theory of impression management to illuminate interprofessional practice on hospital wards. *Social Science and Medicine, 72,* 1595–1602. https://doi.org/10.1016/j.socscimed.2011.03.037.

Milner, P., & Frawley, P. (2018). From 'on' to 'with' to 'by': People with a learning diability creating a space for the third wave of inclusive research. *Qualitative Research.* https://doi.org/10.1177/1468794118781385.

Pollock, K. (2012). Procedure versus process: Ethical paradigms and the conduct of qualitative research. *BMC Medical Ethics, 13*(1), 25.

Salmon, G. (2013). *E-tivities: The key to active online learning.* New York and London: Routledge.

Sanjari, M., Bahramnezhad, F., Fomani, F. K., Shoghi, M., & Cheraghi, M. A. (2014). Ethical challenges of researchers in qualitative studies: The necessity to develop a specific guideline. *Journal of Medical Ethics and History of Medicine, 7,* 14–20.

Stevenson, F. A., Gibson, W., Pelletier, C., Chrysikou, V., & Park, S. (2015). Reconsidering 'ethics' and 'quality' in healthcare research: The case for an iterative ethical paradigm. *BMC Medical Ethics, 16*(1), 21.

Part II

Identifying and Understanding the Complexities of MDT Meetings

4

Theorising Multidisciplinary Team Meetings in Mental Health Clinical Practice

Cordet Smart and Timothy Auburn

Introduction

In this chapter, we seek to examine in more detail the implications for multidisciplinary team meetings of adopting an 'emic' discursive approach to their functioning. In Chapter 2, we set out the conversation analytic (CA) approach adopted as our main methodology throughout this book. Three main principles of CA were described: turn taking, sequence organisation and repair. Through the application of these principles to instances of health care interactions, it was shown how the organisation of those interactions could be described and also how that organisation displayed for the participants the interpersonal projects that they were pursuing (e.g. optimising health care outcomes).

C. Smart (✉) · T. Auburn
School of Psychology, University of Plymouth, Plymouth, UK
e-mail: cordet.smart@plymouth.ac.uk

T. Auburn
e-mail: T.Auburn@plymouth.ac.uk

© The Author(s) 2018
C. Smart and T. Auburn (eds.), *Interprofessional Care and Mental Health*,
The Language of Mental Health, https://doi.org/10.1007/978-3-319-98228-1_4

Here, we want to extend that analysis specifically to interactions during multidisciplinary team meetings and consider what projects members are pursuing and to what extent the team meeting context enables members to pursue such projects.

The Context of Team Meetings

Our first point is self-evident. First and foremost team meetings are meetings. They are not casual encounters between friends, they are not sitting with a patient and explaining a care plan, and they are not corridor interactions between doctors and nurses out of sight of patients on a ward (Lewin & Reeves, 2011). They are formal, organisationally constituted encounters between several people with different disciplinary backgrounds and an agenda of topics to be covered within a set time.

The range of encounters listed above would normally be regarded as arising from different sorts of social context. It is the context which gives meaning to the encounter and allows its participants to understand what the motives and concerns of each other are. Conversation analysis has a particular approach to conceptualising context which differs in many respects from conventional psychological or sociological understandings. The conventional way of conceptualising context is to regard it as a social framework which shapes the interaction that occurs within it. Thus a court of law, a doctor's surgery or a classroom each shape or constrain, in particular ways, the sorts of actions that go on within them. This conceptualisation of context is a 'top-down' one.

In contrast, conversation analysis conceptualises context as 'bottom up'; more formally, context is 'endogenously' constituted (Heritage, 1984). By this phrase is meant that the context and all its meanings, rights, obligations, identities of participants and so on are not externally given or imposed but are accomplished and oriented to through the activities of the actors themselves on a turn-by-turn basis.

Sidnell (2010) has outlined the conversational 'machinery' through which context is endogenously constituted. First, the very sequential organisation of turns of talk creates a context for a next positioned turn. Adjacency pairs, for example, are a widespread way of organising talk (see Chapter 2), and the first and second parts of adjacency pairs are type related; issuing a first pair part will create the context for the relevance of a particular second pair part. Moreover, participants to a conversation make their contribution to the interaction, topic-relevant and designed for the particular recipient or recipients of their talk and in doing so, participants display their understanding of the context and the roles and identities of the other participants. This account of how context is constituted is often treated as an account of the micro-context. So how is the macro-context, those social institutions which are regarded as the forming the texture of society, such as class, gender, ethnicity, and their associated identities, constituted? Sidnell argues that the 'macro-context' is constituted in much the same way as the micro-context.

From a 'top-down' perspective, in claiming that a social institution creates a context which shapes people's actions, the analyst is selecting a description of that setting from the many possible descriptions available and asserting its relevance to the actions of the participants. Conversation analysts, however, insist that the analyst making such an assertion needs to demonstrate the relevance and the 'procedural consequentiality' of that characterisation of the context for the participants themselves. The way in which this relevance is demonstrated is in the progressivitiy of the interaction through the design of turns of talk. Thus, it is in the design of turns of talk and the progressive development of the interaction through these turns that 'the context' gets established and maintained as a cooperative accomplishment of the participants. The interaction order, the systematically organised domain of face-to-face interaction, as defined by Goffman (1983), therefore underlies the operation of all other 'macro' social institutions.

Any particular social institution is constituted by its members through their orientation to the relevance of that particular characterisation of it. It follows that there must be something in the way people engage with one another that displays that for them they are participating in that particular institution. For example is there something in the way that a doctor and patient design their turns of talk and manage their engagement with one another which displays for them that, at that moment and for all practical purposes, they are taking part in a GP consultation? For conversation analysts, the answer to this question is a clear affirmative.

The organisation of informal everyday conversation is taken as the baseline for all other types of encounters. How people conduct themselves in other institutional contexts occur as systematic adaptations of this baseline. For example in a court of law, it is notable how this institution is constituted, inter alia, out of a variation of question and answer sequences which have their foundation in such sequences in informal conversation. The design of these sequences in turn displays the relevant roles and their associated rights and obligations, for example, the lawyer who has the right to ask questions and the witness who is obliged to answer questions. This is not to argue that participants slavishly follow such norms; within any encounter, there are options in how the participants design their talk in order to manage their projects and identity.

'Meeting Talk'

This diversion into the way that conversation analysis conceptualises context brings us back to our initial observation that team meetings are first and foremost meetings. The proposal that institutional encounters are in an important sense adaptations of the baseline speech exchange system applies therefore to multidisciplinary meetings (Svennevig, 2012). Svennevig (2012) makes the point: "Thus, conducting a meeting means orienting to the normative practices constitutive of this speech exchange system, that is, producing 'meeting talk'" (p. 4). Svennevig (2012) goes on to identify some of the main normative practices to which meeting members orient.

- *'The most distinguishing feature of meeting interaction is the presence of a chair that is charged with managing the access to the floor and assuring the topical progression of the meeting according to the agenda. These tasks provide the chair with special rights and obligations in controlling the contributions of the participants. He or she has a dominating and privileged position in being authorized to encourage contributions and actions that are considered constructive to the goals of the meeting and sanction behaviour that is considered illegitimate or counter-productive. Also, in formulating decisions and conclusions the chair acquires a strategic position in the meeting'* (Svennevig, 2012, p. 5).

- The chair takes the responsibility for allocating turns to members; conversely, members often display their wish to take a speaking turn through various forms of signalling (e.g. nods, 'catching the eye' of the chair). Even where a member specifically selects another member as the next speaker (e.g. I would be interested in hearing x's view on this), the go ahead for x to start speaking is often sanctioned through the chair.

- There is a mix of self-selection and pre-allocation of turns by the chair. *'Sometimes the chair will let speakers self-select as long as the conversation runs smoothly, and only intervene with explicit turn allocation in cases where problems arise, such as unresolved competition for the floor'* (Svennevig, 2012, p. 6).

- Multimodal practices are frequent, and the types of practices are well established and mutually understood (e.g. pointing as a speaker selection practice, catching the eye of the chair).

- There is usually a written agenda as a way of specifying topic(s) in advance.

- As with many institutional settings, formulations (Heritage & Watson, 1979) are a device used by participants to gain agreement of the other co-present members and to progress the agenda item under discussion. A specific practice utilised by chairs is to issue 'candidate pre-closing formulations' (Barnes, 2007). Such formulations achieve a display of the orderliness of the prior discussion and provide a slot for further discussion as a next turn, although the norm as a second part is silence. Silence displays the other member's agreement with the formulation and leads smoothly into the next topic or agenda item.

- There is usually a range of ways of marking transitions to new agenda item/topic.

- There is often pre-allocation of turns according to agenda items which in turn often entails longer, monological turns.

- Turns are often less tied to an immediately previous contribution but oriented to positioning of turn in the sequence through introductory prefaces.
- Meetings are often characterised by the multimodal use of devices or other artefacts (PowerPoint presentations, papers, other documents or diagrams).
- Members have resources for moving in and out of meeting talk (Deppermann, Schmitt, & Mondada, 2010).
- Meetings are multiparty encounters, hence making more salient the need for coordination of contributions and for achieving the aims for which the meeting was convened.

It is through the orientation to and performance of these (and other practices), which are recognisably adaptations of informal conversational practices, that organisations are 'talked into being'. Further, meetings are where organisational culture and knowledge is created, negotiated and disseminated and where organisational roles and relations are manifested (Svennevig, 2012). It is at this level of 'mundane' collaboration between members of teams that the broader principle of 'interprofessional working' will be constituted and negotiated. To paraphrase Ervin Goffman, it is the mundane interaction order of the meeting that underpins the production of the institutional order of interprofessional working.

MDTs and Meeting Talk

Meeting talk, then, can be considered to 'bring into being' the organisation. It also represents a particular form of interactional practice, through which MDTs are able to act. Within the constraints of the meeting talk, then, we can also observe the effects of the constitution of MDT meetings for how members orientate to their institutional concerns and display these in their meeting interactions.

One of the points made in Chapter 2 was that there was evidence for a 'problematic disjuncture' in so far as there is a discrepancy between the aspiration for interprofessional working and the way in which it is actually implemented in multidisciplinary team meetings. The normative practices characterising meeting talk outlined in the previous section suggest some of the ways in which this disjuncture may come about.

- An absence of the relevant personnel from the meeting. Lewin and Reeves (2011) identified that doctors and nurses in their observational study infrequently attended MDT meetings and that the absence of doctors hindered decision making around patient discharges. This observation suggests that the team members were oriented to interprofessional participation in case decisions and that doctors' and nurses' absence was a breach of these normative expectations and so an accountable absence. Indeed, the doctors and nurses interviewed in their study displayed extensive 'no fault' accounting for their absence.
- The style or manner in which chairs of meetings implement their chairing role. In his review, Svennevig (2012) implies that there are 'hard' and 'soft' ways of doing chairing. For example, '... *there is large room for variation in how strictly the chair will control the topic by reference to the agenda, or allow the topic to be locally managed and possibly drift into adjacent matters*' (p. 7). A chair may also allow members to self-select for a speaking turn or manage the allocation of speaking turns more strictly. Pomerantz and Denvir (2007) found that when a chair occupied a non-senior position, they presented themselves as a 'facilitator' and was more likely to ask the other members' opinions about procedure as well as presenting directions to participants as merely suggestions.
- The way in which organisational role and the epistemic authority carried by that role is enacted in the meeting. Lewin and Reeves (2011) observed ward rounds and suggested that professionals other than doctors had a peripheral role and that the performance of a ward round was ritualistic perpetuating medical dominance in health care. In a similar setting, Arber (2008) found that in order for nurses to make a medical contribution, in the presence of consultant doctors, to an MDT they adopted a strategic form of question asking marked by various pre-expansions which displayed the delicacy of initiating

their question. She attributes this practice as occasioned by an orientation to their lower medical status *vis-à-vis* medical doctors.

In what follows we provide some exemplars of how MDT meetings were interactionally constituted in our project and how an orientation to interprofessional working may be discernible in the activities of the meeting members.

Project Overview

This project was based on an analysis of management meetings in services which supported people with intellectual disabilities (Intellectual (Learning) Disability [I(L)D] Services). As with the other studies within this book, the project involved the recording and analysis of team meetings that were held within this service. For this part of the project, the focus was on 12 hours of team meetings comprising four different meetings. The process of seeking permission to record as well as undertaking the recording of the meetings themselves was our first opportunity to develop our understanding of interprofessional working in the particular context of multidisciplinary team meetings.

First, it seemed appropriate to gain an understanding of the specific background that was relevant to the working of these teams. We did this through conversations with service users (see also Chapter 13) and clinicians, as well as undertaking literature reviews so that we could gain an insight into the challenges for the health professionals of working within these teams. Based on a thematic analysis, four types of concern which members brought to meetings were identified:

- local service needs,
- the broader political context,
- professional similarities and differences
- and interpersonal concerns, such as friendships.

We used these our understanding of these concerns to orient us to an analysis of the data, in particular, how these operated in the context of the MDT meeting. Our general analytic strategy was an iterative one, where we examined the details of the interactions, and then considered how these interactional particulars might fit with the range of concerns articulated by those with a stake in the outcomes of the meetings.

The Context of I(L)D MDT Meetings

Our observations identified the key features of the MDT meetings: members have particular roles that are designated, sometimes only at the point that the members assemble, that there was a pre-circulated agenda, that there was a set time and location for the meeting, and that normally members sat in a circle, often around a central desk. The meetings from which extracts are reported comprised between 8 and 12 people.

The audio-recording tape was turned on at the beginning of the meeting as people were still assembling. Once members were settled, the meeting was formally opened by the chair. The first business was considering apologies, acceptance of the minutes from the last meeting and prior action points. Each agenda point was then considered in turn, before the meeting was brought to a close by the chair. Thus, a very particular organisation for interactions was established commensurate with the range of practices identified above for organisational meetings in general.

The Role of the Chair

The following example (Extract 1, see also Chapter 2) illustrates the canonical role of the chair in effecting a transition from one agenda point to the next. This example illustrates the unproblematic display of mundane collaboration between the meeting members.

Extract 1: Transition from One Agenda Point to the Next
(C2: 0:01:52:21-0:02:01:52
San: Meeting chair; Car: Meeting member)

```
1   San:      >Are you happy with the< accuracy:: ↑=

2   Car:      =Yep. Fine.

3   San:      >Any further amendment:s (.)  ↑then<apart

4             from Jon Taylor:s ↑

5             Good Oka:y↓ °let' s move on°
```

In line 1, Sandra's turn is an interrogatively designed first pair part. It can be heard as a pre-closing request referencing the preceding talk and therefore as the opening of a move into closure of that agenda item. Typical of such requests, it is also designed so that the preferred response is an affirmative. Although it doesn't have an explicit pro-term, it implicitly operates to connect to the prior talk. This formulation produces an affirmative from Caroline (line 2: yep) which is immediately upgraded with a 'fine'.

Although one of team members has supplied a relevant second pair part, Sandra nevertheless at line 3 pursues affiliation from the team members. At first sight, it is a puzzle as to why she feels the need to pursue a further receipt of her request, after all there appears to be consensus agreement as voiced by Caroline. One answer comes from the work of Barnes (2007) on pre-closing formulations. In her analysis of multi-professional education teams, Barnes identified that the preferred second to such formulations from the chair is no response or silence. The fact that Caroline has responded, albeit with an affirmative, may provide for the inference that there is some disagreement or problem with this formulation. Sandra reissues her interrogative, but it has noticeably changed its content. It repairs her prior turn by now acknowledging that an amendment is needed and who the author of that amendment is. The reissued formulation is in a declarative format but with a rising intonation at the end of the TCU (indicated by the up arrow on 'then') and a negative interrogative term ('any'). This design reverses the polarity of the interrogative so that the preferred response is now disconfirmation. The response on this occasion is silence (end of line 4), which according to Barnes is the preferred response indicating agreement and so gives the go ahead for Sandra as chair to mark the transition to a new agenda item (line 5).

In terms of marking this move into the next item, Sandra delivers a positive evaluation—'good' in line 5, followed by 'Okay' and then 'let's move on'. This three-part transition, evaluation + Okay + a move on statement, was repeatedly used to close an agenda point and prepare the ground for the next. It appears to construct a level of agreement for the meeting members that permits the chair to move the meeting to the next agenda point. These transition practices were generally preceded by a closing sequence (Schegloff, 2007), seen here in the pre-closing request in line 1.

This transition is particularly rapid compared with other CA studies of agenda-orientated talk, such as Deppermann et al. (2010). Noticeably, staff repeatedly commented on the time pressures on these meetings, the costs of so many high-level staff meeting together and their pride in achieving the organisational task requirements in a timely fashion. Thus, the design of these closings and openings seems attuned to local service priorities, concerns with time management and could be considered collaborative in the sense that they were not resisted by meeting members.

Inserting Queries and Flexible Chairing

In Extract 1, it was noted how the chair engages in a recognisable practice with which the other team members collaborate to produce a closing of one agenda item and a smooth transition to a new agenda item. The following extract shows this same practice, but here it is resisted by one of the team members. This resistance displays at an interpersonal level how members design their turns to sustain a collaborative orientation to one another. It also displays the sort of concerns that members bring to the meeting and which animate their agreement or not with the decisions that are a main purpose of the meeting.

Extract 2: Resisting Moving On

(C1:32.43.3-33:28.3
San: Chair; Sal: Other team member)

```
1  San:      >okay↓ lovely↓<right now< emm are eye [MRI]

2            ↓scans procedures<right we we

3            >can take that< off now

4  Sal:      is that sorted

5  San:      I thi:nk, Richard was going<to go

6            go awa<do you know anything ↑about th:at,
```

In line 1, Sandra, the chair, marks a transition to a new agenda
item ('okay lovely right' + new item) and immediately goes on to propose removing that next item from the meeting agenda (lines 2–3: we
can take that off now). It is delivered as a declarative without any of
the intonational features which would make this an interrogative. It
therefore functions as a proposed course of action, which would normally elicit agreement as the preferred second. If it was agreed, then it
would allow a further moving on to the next agenda item. However, the
assumed implicit team agreement is challenged by Sally at line 4 where
she asks: 'is that sorted'. This can be heard as a dispreferred response to
the chair's declarative but delivered using an interrogative format; this in
turn resists the chair's projected course of action of closing this agenda
item and moving to the next.

There are two features of Sally's turn in line 4 which are noteworthy. First, the turn is delivered as an interrogative. Although this can
be heard as a dispreferred second, it also is designed neither to affiliate nor to disaffiliate with the course of action the chair has proposed.
This interrogative format is similar to the practice identified by Arber
(2008) where question asking was a practice which allowed nurses as
team members to make proposals from a position of lower epistemic
authority. Here, Sally by designing her intervention as an interrogative

positions herself as epistemically lower status and therefore seeking information which will inform her. This intervention is designed to register a concern about the issue but by neither affiliating nor disaffiliating is also attentive to the maintenance of social relations within the team.

The second feature of this intervention is that it displays Sally's concern with the wider institutional service provision being discussed. This questioning by Sally registers a concern around service provision of MRI procedures for people with I(L)D, opening the floor for discussion. This question could be heard as resistant to the course of action proposed by the chair. However, by re-framing our understanding of the question as introducing a concern about service provision, it can be heard as legitimate. Indeed, the question is not treated as problematic here. It is not dismissed and does not cause any lapses. Instead, that particular concern is re-prioritised by the chair. Above we identified that how a chair implements their role can vary on a continuum from informal to formal. The chair here displays flexibility in allowing this agenda item to develop as a discussion. The chair initially attempts an answer to this question, which is marked by some uncertainty (I think, line 5) and then abandoned (line 6), in favour of allocating the next turn to Richard who is (presumably) knowledgeable enough to provide an adequate answer.

The 'Same' Community

Our third example displays one of the ways in which chairs orient to the team as an institutional unit. One common method for identifying individuals as members of the same community is the use of the institutional 'we' (Drew & Heritage, 1992). There is an example of this use in Extract 1 (line 5) and Extract 2 (line 2). The practice we draw attention to in this example is the use of laughter as an affiliative device which constitutes the team as an in-group in contrast to others outside the group.

Extract 3: Laughter as an Affiliative Device

(C2:1:38:50.1-1:39:06.4
Sue: team member; Bob: team member: San: chair)

```
1  Sue:      the rest of us wi:ll >↑but not

2            the £new manager£

3  Bob:      yea [yes

4  Sue:          [↑he he hu ↓hu

5            (0.8)

6  San:      oka:y let' s move on↓ six point tw:o↓

7            COUNS
```

This extract comes at the end of a discussion of how things might change with a new manager who has recently joined the service. Sue begins to transform the prior agenda point into a laughable by using a contrast organisation indicated by the contrastive connective (but) and speaking with a smiley voice 'not the £new manager£' in the second component. Agreement tokens are then provided by Bob in line 3 which affiliates with Sue's smiley voice. Affirming laughter follows in line 4, with the downward intonation indicating a closing of the prior agenda point. This is followed by a lapse in the conversation (line 5). Sandra self-selects, as is the right invested in the chair and initiates a transition to a new agenda item (lines 6–7: Okay + move on + new item).

Laughter can initiate interpersonal collaboration (Glenn, 2003) and has been considered as important for interprofessional working (Griffiths, 1998). The other feature of this exchange is the use by Sue of the institutional 'we', which is set up in contrast to the 'new manager'. The use of 'we' and the mention of the 'new manager' as a laughable are oriented to constituting the team members as part of the same community.

Summary and Conclusions

In this chapter, we have focused on multidisciplinary team meetings as first and foremost meetings. We have explored what implications participation in that mode of interprofessional working has for those who are required to work in that way. Initially, we outlined the CA conceptualisation of context as a corrective to the view that context has a determining or shaping effect on the actions that occur in that setting. The position that contexts are endogenously constituted was then outlined. The practices which are resources for endogenously constituting meetings as particular contexts were then delineated. We suggested that some of the problems associated with the poor implementation of interprofessional working in team meetings could be understood by reference to these practices.

Furthermore, these practices can be regarded as contributing to 'mundane' collaboration between participants in pursuing and achieving their projects. Through the analysis of selected examples, we have then attempted to illustrate how the wider institutional concerns emerge from and are oriented to through this mundane collaboration. Specifically, these examples demonstrated that the chair and the other members of the team, through recognisable meeting-specific practices, achieve the flexible participation of members of the team in discussions of I(L)D issues, as well as the constitution of the participants as members of the same community.

This chapter has presented a tentative first step and focused exclusively on management meetings in order to enable a specific focus on the ways that the institutional orientation to interprofessional working was present throughout the meetings. This potentially offers an 'ideal' form of organisational meeting and was the most institutionalised of all of the meetings that we considered within the study, in that the agenda points and action points were clearly adhered to.

Implications for Interprofessional Working

- It seems important for the chair of meetings to recognise that there are different ways of implementing this role and to consider that a more flexible, open and less formalised approach is more likely to be commensurate with the principles of interprofessional working.
- MDT members should take the opportunity to affirm a positive in-group identity through their interactions in the meeting.

References

Arber, A. (2008). Team meetings in specialist palliative care: Asking questions as a strategy within interprofessional interaction. *Qualitative Health Research, 18*, 1323–1335. https://doi.org/10.1177/1049732308322588.

Barnes, R. (2007). Formulations and the facilitation of common agreement in meetings talk. *Text and Talk, 27*, 273–296. https://doi.org/10.1515/TEXT.2007.011.

Deppermann, A., Schmitt, R., & Mondada, L. (2010). Agenda and emergence: Contingent and planned activities in a meeting. *Journal of Pragmatics, 42*, 1700–1718. https://doi.org/10.1016/j.pragma.2009.10.006.

Drew, P., & Heritage, J. (Eds.). (1992). *Talk at work*. Cambridge: Cambridge University Press.

Glenn, P. J. (2003). *Laughter in interaction*. New York: Cambridge University Press.

Goffman, E. (1983). The interaction order: American sociological association, 1982 presidential address. *American Sociological Review, 48*, 1–17.

Griffiths, L. (1998). Humour as resistance to professional dominance in community mental health teams. *Sociology of Health & Illness, 20*, 874–895.

Heritage, J. (1984). *Garfinkel and ethnomethodology*. Cambridge: Polity Press.

Heritage, J., & Watson, R. (1979). Formulations as conversational objects. In G. Psathas (Ed.), *Everyday language: Studies in ethnomethodology* (pp. 123–162). New York: Irvington.

Lewin, S., & Reeves, S. (2011). Enacting 'team' and 'teamwork': Using Goffman's theory of impression management to illuminate interprofessional practice on hospital wards. *Social Science and Medicine, 72,* 1595–1602. https://doi.org/10.1016/j.socscimed.2011.03.037.

Pomerantz, A., & Denvir, P. (2007). Enacting the institutional role of chairperson in upper management meetings: The interactional realization of provisional authority. In F. Cooren (Ed.), *Interacting and organizing: Analyses of a management meeting* (pp. 31–52). London: Lawrence Erlbaum.

Schegloff, E. A. (2007). *Sequence organization in interaction: A primer in conversation analysis* (Vol. 1). Cambridge: Cambridge University Press.

Sidnell, J. (2010). *Conversation analysis: An introduction.* West Sussex, UK: Wiley-Blackwell.

Svennevig, J. (2012). Interaction in workplace meetings. *Discourse Studies, 14,* 3–10. https://doi.org/10.1177/1461445611427203.

5

Power Struggles in MDT Meetings: Using Different Orders of Interaction to Understand the Interplay of Hierarchy, Knowledge and Accountability

Cordet Smart, Christianne Pollock, Lindsay Aikman and Erica Willoughby

Introduction

The literature review presented in Chapter 1 identified a range of organisational features which affect how MDTs operate. This chapter focuses on one of those features, namely the effects of power and professional hierarchies. Power struggles are a major concern in many (if not all) interactional contexts. John Heritage (e.g. 2012) has

C. Smart (✉)
School of Psychology, University of Plymouth, Plymouth, UK
e-mail: cordet.smart@plymouth.ac.uk

C. Pollock
NHS England, Transforming Care Programme, London, UK
e-mail: nezumi3@me.com

L. Aikman
Livewell Southwest, Plymouth, UK
e-mail: lindsay.aikman@nhs.net

conducted a considerable amount of work on power from a conversation analytic perspective focusing on what he terms epistemic authority, the way in which claims to particular sorts of knowledge constitute an entitlement for a certain course of action to prevail over a potential other course of action. The MDT meeting is no different—there are inherent power struggles, not always dramatic, but certainly present in the subtle negotiation of authority to make decisions. In the MDT context, these negotiations are framed by organisational and professional hierarchies, and limited staff time. The broad model of MDTs, as discussed in Chapters 1 and 2, implies that at least part of their purpose is for the voices of multiple professionals to be heard and for every member to contribute equally to decision making. This aim has challenged the traditional hierarchies frequently found both within healthcare organisations and between professionals (Baker, Egan-Lee, Martimianakis, & Reeves, 2011; Gair & Hartery, 2001; McCallin, 1999). Indeed the power differentials that exist between professionals can present the most significant challenge to interprofessional working (see Chapter 1 and Reeves et al., 2009). Collaborative team working arguably requires a more egalitarian approach; shared planning and decision-making; shared responsibility throughout the team; non-hierarchical relationships in the team; and shared power as a result of individual knowledge and expertise (Henneman, Lee, & Cohen, 1995).

This chapter explores issues of power within MDTs and, via a project that explored such practices, seeks to extend our knowledge of how power works in MDTs at an interactional level.

Definitions of Power

We argue that it would be a mistake to accept a single definition of power, and potentially unhelpful for understanding how it operates in the MDT meeting. To help us to better understand power,

E. Willoughby
Cornwall Partnership NHS Foundation Trust, Cornwall, UK
e-mail: erica.willoughby@nhs.net

here we summarise the position of Pratto (2015), who published a landmark paper in the *British Journal of Social Psychology* that summarised current perspectives and debates on power. She proposed that power is fundamental to understanding multiple contexts due to, among other things, its relevance to morality, negative outcomes such as domination, and positive effects when used conjointly to achieve group aims. She discussed key debates and transitions in the historical understanding of power. Most significantly, she highlighted a transition from understanding power as a property of a person or object, to viewing it as relational or constructed between people. This approach recognises that any influence of personality traits is mediated in complex ways by situational and personal factors. This represents a change in our understanding of power—earlier historical approaches focused more on personality. She suggests this change can be attributed to schools of thought such as Social Identity Theory (SIT) (Haslam, Reicher, & Platow, 2011; Turner, 1990) and Leader Membership Exchange (LMX) theory (Gerstner & Day, 1997), where the focus has been on the *relationship* between the leader and the followers. Understandings of leadership and power developed from SIT highlight group effects. For example, a leader might emerge from a group because they represent prototypical properties of the group. Consequently, followers give the person power.

Leader membership exchange theory is based on the assumption that the basis of power in leadership is through bargaining and exchange between leaders and subordinates. Personality factors affecting how people are leaders or followers then become secondary to the relationship itself (Yoon & Bono, 2016). Further, Pratto (2015) discusses how we can differentiate 'power over' and 'power to'. 'Power to' reflects the degree to which a person can achieve their own goals—akin to empowerment principles. 'Power over' is the capacity to direct others. In both cases, power can be seen as having the ability to meet personal goals or the goals of others, to have agency over self and/or others. Power therefore should be considered as a complex construct. It is likely that all of these ways of conceptualising power are negotiated and labelled as 'power' in lay discussions of how meetings work, without the subtle distinctions proposed by researchers.

Pratto also highlighted the frequent assumption that power is inherently bad—but in many cases power over someone can be a necessity. For example, the power of a carer for their loved one is not always bad. To have the power to care can be healthy, for example a carer of a person with a learning disability might enable that person to have access to services by directing them to the relevant contact. Thus, the power to influence and to be influenced within an MDT meeting needs careful consideration and reflection.

Think point

 Power often needs unpacking to really understand its complexity. It can be understood as:

1. Ability to do different things: e.g. access resources, influence people.
2. Power can take different forms—knowledge, emotional, social.
3. Power can be given through social structures or a person might choose to take control.

Power and Hierarchies in Mental Health Settings

Definitions of power within mental health settings often appear to reflect 'power over'. Research has tended to focus on the effects of organisational or professional hierarchies, rather than individual agency. Further, the possible negative connotations of power are often raised. There seems to be a complex interplay between perceptions of who has power over whom, the traditional medical hierarchy and the professional training available to MDT teams. As we developed this brief review, it became increasingly clear that any attempt at disentangling these relationships might not represent effectively the contexts of MDT working (see Chapter 4 for further discussion of context and meeting talk). We suggest that this further supports Pratto's (2015) assertion of the essential consideration of power as a series of personal relationships, as a social construct, rather than as a feature of personality.

At an organisational level, the UK's National Health Service (NHS) has traditionally operated with a clearly defined hierarchical structure (Klein, 1982). This structure assigns some members of staff more 'power over' than is assigned to others (Baker et al., 2011; Currie, Lockett, Finn, Martin, & Waring, 2012). Within mental health contexts, this assignment of 'power over' is often to the psychiatrist. Other staff, such as psychologists, are typically thought to hold 'expert power' related to their profession and have been seen to 'chip in' to MDT meetings (Christofides, Johnstone, & Musa, 2012) in relation to their professional experience. In contrast, psychiatrists or managers' views are often considered more pervasive throughout decisions and meetings (Lipman, 2000). These implicit rules of who might have power seem to be adhered to by lesser powerful (e.g. support workers) and more powerful clinicians (e.g. medical consultants). Indeed, highly trained clinicians can assume that they should be at the top of the hierarchical system in order to reflect the training they have undertaken (Baker et al., 2011). The resulting effect is that 'highly trained' staff, such as medical doctors, clinical psychologists and nurse specialists, have more power over than 'lesser trained', such as junior nurses or support workers (Marriott, 2008). In summary, the hierarchical structure means that clinicians with professional level training can exert greater 'power over', though this might be done in different ways—generic if they are a psychiatrist, or 'expert specific' if they are of another profession, than those with no professional level qualification.

Although it might seem obvious, or even appropriate, that those with greater qualification should have more influence, what can happen is that the perspective of others, such as those who know the service users better, might remain unheard negatively affecting interprofessional working and leaving services at risk of poorer practice (see Chapter 1, 2). For example, a hierarchical structure supporting differentiation between physicians and non-physicians can be detrimental for team working and prevent collaborative decision-making (Cott, 1997, 1998). Heritage (2012), discussing work by Anspach (1993), uses the example of neonatal intensive care units, where despite the nurses' 'extended and textured' knowledge of babies in their care, decisions may be made by consultant doctors that rely on readings from patients charts, rather than being informed by the nursing staff. Nevertheless, it has been possible to overcome some of these issues where the hierarchical system is one of professional respect as opposed to perceived elevation of power (Crosby, 2010). Problematically, however, this results in those staff with less training who often have the most contact time with service users (Butler et al., 2018) not being able to contribute to the same extent. It has been found that members of staff lower in the hierarchical structure make fewer contributions in an MDT setting (Maddock, 2014; Oborn & Dawson, 2010; Reeves et al., 2009; Rowlands & Callen, 2013) and more support is needed to promote involvement from these individuals (Atwal & Caldwell, 2005). It is recognition of these issues that has encouraged changes to the MDT model, such that thought is given about how power may be shared and how decision-making may be achieved, such that all voices can be heard.

There are a range of issues around power that are specific to MDT working. The MDT is often structured in ways that mirror the hierarchical structure traditionally observed in healthcare settings (Ogland-Hand & Zeiss, 2000), thus challenging their effectiveness as locations for interprofessional locations. Thus, the differential in influence on decisions and discussions is also mirrored (Propp et al., 2010). However, there is limited research exploring how to train MDTs to function in a more supportive and collaborative way (Janss, Rispens, Segers, & Jehn, 2012). Some have argued that power in MDTs is a finite resource (Weber, Lukes, & Webb, 1986), and for collaboration to take place it needs to be evenly distributed. Power differentials occurring in MDTs are described as creating power struggles (Johnson, 2009), in turn creating less safe practice in part due to poorer communication between staff (Nadzam, 2009), with worse patient outcomes (Marshall & Robson, 2005), and less team engagement, limiting interprofessional learning and involvement (Currie, Finn, & Martin, 2010; Currie & Suhomlinova, 2006).

Arguably, part of the change inherent in MDTs in moving towards interprofessional working is also ensuring clear accountability. A central change to clinical practice within MDTs is around 'shared' vs 'professional' responsibility, and so the sharing of power might also relate to a sharing of responsibility (Koeck, 2014), which may create tensions for interprofessional working. Dunne, Jaffar, and Latoo (2013) critique these new ways of working and discuss the need for MDTs to be properly managed and not 'rudderless', so that accountability and responsibility for risk is unclear. It might be that this lack of clarity around power and responsibility leads to more complex power struggles in MDT working. Thus, in line with Pratto's (2015) perspective, the construction of power seems very much relational, between professionals, and also very much situated within a particular discursive tapestry of responsibility and hierarchy.

Power and Conversation Analysis

To tease out the relational aspects of power and the ways that it is negotiated in MDT meetings, we used the constructs of epistemics and deontics (Stevanovic & Peräkylä, 2014). We intended that a bottom-up analysis would help to tease out power struggles, exploring power relationships as interactional in line with Pratto (2015). Rather than evaluating power as either good or bad, we wished to explore how it works in practice. Both epistemics and deontics have been studied in terms of conflict management and information sharing in conversations (Landmark, Gulbrandsen, & Svennevig, 2015; Stevanovic & Peräkylä, 2012). Each is briefly described.

Epistemic order (authority) is concerned with individual speaker's rights and *access to knowledge* (Raymond & Heritage, 2006). Professionals bring different areas of expertise to MDTs. Within the MDT, these different knowledge statuses will be reflected both in talk design and also in how others respond. Understanding of others' actions comes from an ongoing assessment of our knowledge and that of others in the team (Heritage, 2012).

Heritage (2012) makes a distinction between a person's epistemic status—derived from outside of the immediate interaction—and their epistemic stance—the position that a person takes within the interaction. The degree of knowledge or understanding an individual has can be described as ranging from shallow to deep (Heritage, 2010; Heritage

& Raymond, 2012) which in turn relates to a lower or higher epistemic status, respectively (Heritage, 2012). Epistemic status fluctuates throughout a conversation according to each individual's specialism, or epistemic domain (area of knowledge) (Heritage, 2012). Claims to 'knowing more' give an individual greater authority in interactions and make them less likely to be challenged. When MDTs have been purposely developed to share responsibility for decision-making, it is essential that there is mutual understanding within the team regarding the knowledge bases of the different participants and also their role within that team. This allows for effective collaboration as relevant information can be gathered from those with the knowledge to provide it. Orientation towards epistemic order rather than hierarchy provides an opportunity for those with the most appropriate knowledge to contribute.

Think point

 Epistemic order is the way in which people orient to knowledge:

1. The epistemic status of different professionals within the MDT will vary depending upon the topic under discussion.
2. The epistemic stance adopted by a speaker is not always consistent with their epistemic status. People choose how to design their talk to reflect their stance.
3. Institutions may ascribe different epistemic rights to people in different roles.

Deontic order (authority) is related to the rights and obligations of the speaker to *influence actions* related to the conversation (Stevanovic & Peräkylä, 2012). Deontic claims can lead to deontic congruence, where the future action is accepted, or deontic incongruence, where the suggestion is resisted. Power, authority and therefore deontic and epistemic rights are not absolute. Deontic order varies between different domains and a person may have more right to decide about future actions in some domains when compared to others.

Deontic order relates to how an individual's actions may prohibit another individual from participating in a certain way, or continuing with a course of action. Deontic stance and status can also be distinguished, and again, shift through interactions. The relationship between deontic order and obligations means that deontic order is aligned with responsibilities. Within mental health settings, the deontic stance displayed by a speaker may be expected to reflect the responsibilities and accountability of that person.

The deontic rights of an MDT member may vary depending on their role in a particular MDT. For example, in the UK in some contexts the psychiatrist acts as a 'Responsible Clinician', where they take on a formal, legal role of responsibility and are as an individual held accountable when a person does not have capacity to decide a future course of action. Their position within an MDT might be quite different, where responsibility is shared. In cases of shared responsibility, we may expect to see this dilution of deontic rights expressed through the talk.

Think point

 Deontic order is related to the rights and obligations of the speaker to influence actions related to the conversation:

1. The deontic status of professionals within the MDT will vary depending on their role within that MDT.
2. In MDTs with shared responsibility, there will be a dilution of individual deontic rights.

Project Overview

This study aimed to identify power practices in MDT team meetings and to explore how these might affect the interactions and potentially decision-making. A total of 12 hours of team meeting data was used, namely form allocation meetings within two different teams, both of which were from community learning disability services.

Following orthographic transcription, collections were developed of examples where there appeared to be some form of claim to power or authority. These extracts identified points where epistemic and/or deontic claims seemed to be being made. For example, where a person's opinion was heard and accepted by the group, or where an opinion was rejected. About 45 events were collected. Any queries about the extracts were discussed within the wider *MDTsInAction* research group. This provided an opportunity to seek clarity on both the interpretation of data and checking transcription accuracy. It was sometimes difficult to decide whether an excerpt was a power struggle or not, in which case it was rejected.

Findings

We found that power, when considered as epistemic status/stance or deontic status/stance was subtly displayed and taken from different members of the MDT in line with how staff seemed most able to meet the needs of the service user under discussion. For example, when their talk was relevant to the service user's needs then a person would be treated as having greater epistemic or deontic status or stance. The teams used in these examples help us to demonstrate how respect for each other's epistemic status or stance can be implemented, as well as how those who might ostensibly be considered as most powerful in the room if a hierarchical model was considered can also be managed by the group to remove that power.

Respectful Engagement with Each Others Contributions—'Expert Power'?

Extract 1 is taken from an assessment team meeting. It illustrates how a professional might take an 'expert' position in areas that they are professionally trained in, and how these can be respected within interactions. The discussion is of a service user where physical health concerns have been raised by the nurse introducing the service user, and mobility is then discussed by the physiotherapist.

Extract 1

CHR (community nurse and chair of meeting), PHY (physiotherapist), OT (occupational therapist), SLT (speech and language therapist). Also present in the meeting were assistant practitioner, minute taker and psychiatrist.

```
1      PHY:  well >if ↑he's< (0.4) diplegic >which it< sounds
2            li:ke, (0.4) the::n (.) >↑when you get< ↑o:lder you
3            still have quite a lot of upper body strength [but]=
4      CHR:                                               [↑oh]
5      PHY:  =>maybe really< ↑stiff ↑le:gs,=
6      OT:   =↑mm[::]
7      PHY:     [↑b]ut also a risk of hip dislocation,
8      CHR:  n↑yea::h (0.6) I ↑think ↑that was what I was worried
9            abou:t >it ↑just< looked a little pre↑carious (0.4)
10           to ↑me:
11     OT:   [°↑ye:::::s°]
12     SLT:  [↑what's di]plegic then >when you< don't have
13           any:::, (0.4) °movements in [your ↑le:gs?°]
14     PHY:                             [.hhh °ju::st°] just
15           legs are more affected than, (.) than ↑a::rms,
16     CHR:  ↑mm,
17     PHY:  >but they're< (.) ↑usually people who have always
18           got a↑rou:nd independently: and then you ↑get (.)
19           you know you ↑reach (0.4) sixty or what↑ever (0.4)
20           it's  really really stiff legs
```

```
21      SLT:   °↑mm°

22      CHR:   ↓mm::

23             (3.2)

24      PHY:   so ↑does ↑the:, (0.4) have a manua:::l (0.4)

25             ↑wheelchair

26      CHR:   .hhh got an electric ↓wheelchair

27      PHY:   ↓oh right
```

We see in lines 1–3, 5 the physiotherapist provides a claim to epistemic stance (and status) to understand the concerns of the service user. The assessment is prefaced by 'well', which can indicate an elongated turn. The assessment uses technical language to explain likely mobility difficulties. Indications that this authority is accepted come in line 4, where the information is receipted with 'Oh' a newsmark receipt. The physiotherapist continues, and the OT includes minimal continuers in line 6. In line 10 the chair adds their position as an observation of how it was 'to me'. The 'to me' seems to take ownership of an epistemic domain accessible only to her (of her personal observations). This seems to align with the physiotherapist's observations and does not challenge her, though neither support—it might clarify the boundary of the chair's knowledge as a nurse. The physiotherapist continues in line 7 with the SLT in line 12 asking a knowledge-based question of the physiotherapist, which further appears to raise the physiotherapist's epistemic stance in this case. The physiotherapist's answer to this is not challenged but is receipted with minimal acknowledgements. The physiotherapist is then themselves able to take over authority to direct the discussion asking of the chair in lines 24 and 25 what type of wheelchair he has, which the chair responds to. We argue that this extract illustrates the ways that epistemic status and stance can be accepted in a respectful manner within the team, and illustrates potentially an awareness of the boundaries between professions, whilst simultaneously demonstrating interprofessional care.

High Hierarchical but Low Epistemic Status— Management of the Psychiatrist

The next example (Extract 2) is of the psychiatrist attempting unsuccessfully to gain the floor and be heard within a discussion of a service user. Despite his ostensible 'high hierarchical' status, he is treated as if he has low epistemic stance—that is, low knowledge of the service user in this case—and this seems to provide a justification for not giving him space to be heard. Prior to Extract 2 the team have finished discussing a service user, 'Nathan'. They then announce a new service user 'Nicholas Green' and discuss a number of concerns in quick succession relating to his setting and current presentation.

Extract 2: Group Power and Epistemic Status/Stance

CHR (community nurse and chair), MAN (health and social care team manager) PSY (psychiatrist), OT (occupational therapist), SLT (speech and language therapist), SCA (social care assessor), DR (medical doctor). Also present in the meeting were minute taker, primary care liaison nurse and community nurse.

```
1      MAN: this is the la↑ttest (.) ↑isn't ↑i:t?

2      CHR: it ↑is the late[st,]

3      MAN:              [u::]::m,

4      CHR: °°I see (what you mean)°° (0.4) °yea:::h,°

5      PSY: is it na↑than you're talking abou[:t?]

6      MAN:                          [yea]::h ↑tha- no

7           no (0.4) ↑this is nicholas ↓gree::n (0.4) I was just

8           checking ↑nathan's (.) medication he doesn't ↑have

9           medic↑ation (0.4) ↑melatonin's the only natha-

10          e:[r ↑med- medi°cation°]

11     PSY:    [er ↑I'm I'm confu::]::sed ↑u:::::m,

12     ?:   ((blows nose))
```

```
13     PSY:   ↑who ↑is the cha::p ↑who

14     OT:    ↑k'hm hm:::

15     PSY:   who a↑ssaulted people in macdona::lds >is ↑that<

16            nicholas [↑gree::n?]

17     OT:    [↑tha:t's,] [that's [that's nathan]

18     SCA:              [that's [that's nathan]

19     SLT:                      [that's nathan]

20     CHR:              [no:: ↑tha[t's] (.) that's [nathan]

21     MAN:                        [na-]           [that's]

22            nathan [yea::h tha[t's right [yeah yea::h]

23     CHR:          [yeah natha[n,

24     PSY:                      [it ↑wa:s °h[u:::::h hh°]

25     OT:                                   [huh huh huh]

26     CHR:   and ↑nathan's on no medication (.) other than the

27            mela- ↑we:ll he ↑is he's on melatonin

28     MAN:   ↑that's all he's on yea::h (0.6) ↑so, (0.6) ↑u:::m,

29            (0.6) but ↑back to ↑nicholas then

30            (0.8)

31     DR:    °↑oka::y°
```

The extract follows directly the introduction of a new service user, Nicholas Green. The group begin in lines 1–4 with clarification of whether this is the latest information about Nicholas. Their speech is ambiguous: 'this is the latest', for example, and does not specify what information is particularly important. This might reflect a degree of familiarity or shared knowledge already in existence. However, it is clear in line 5 that this is not shared with the psychiatrist, who then asks who they are discussing. In lines 6–10, the manager responds with a clarification and then provides a telling of his actions—that he has checked Nathan's (the prior service user's) information. However, in line 11 the psychiatrist upgrades his query to state that he is confused. His repeated question is acknowledged by the OT in line 14 and is completed in lines 15 and 16. The response is then upgraded by the team in lines 17–25 where five other members of the MDT contribute to clarify that the psychiatrist is referring to Nathan and not the current service user. The manager then repeats the upshot that he previously gave, and they move on. In this extract then, epistemic status/stance seems to be valued above organisational hierarchy in terms of taking control of the meeting.

Group Power—Drowning Out the Psychiatrist

On other occasions, the psychiatrist's input was not considered at all. Again, the majority in the MDT seemed to 'win out'. This time, they simply continued to discuss the service user, without addressing the queries of the psychiatrist. This is exemplified in Extract 3.

Extract 3: Illustrating Group Deontic Status and Stance, and Suppression of Professional Hierarchy

(CHR) community nurse and chair, (MAN) health and social care team manager, (PSY) psychiatrist, (OT) occupational therapist, (SOC) social care assessor. Also present in the meeting were a minute taker, primary care liaison nurse and additional community nurse.

```
1   MAN:    .hhhhh we've go:t (.) um psychology invo:lved (.)

2           ↑he's (.) you know physically

3   CHR:    >I KNOW<

4   MAN:    he's gaining a great deal of w[eight]

5   CHR:                                   [↑yeah]

6   MAN:    his family circumstances are ↑not fantasti:c it's

7           ↑w'll his ↑living situation is not fantast↑i:c and

8           er mm (0.4) he's kinda going nowhe:re (0.4) >in

9           fact< he's getting (0.4) very un↑healthy i- isn't

10          he and he's,

11  PSY:    w- ↑what's his ↑physical health is he something I

12          should ↑↑see:?

13          (1.2)

14  PSY:    cos >you [know< wh- ↑why ↑is ↑he ↑gain]ing so much

15  MAN:             [↑he he was always physically]

16  MAN:    mm:::

17  PSY:    <wei::ght> (.) ↑that, (.) bothers [me] because

18  you=

19  CHR:                                      [mm]

20  PSY:    =kno:::w u:m (0.4) it doesn't ↑have to be
```

```
21              necessarily <due to hi::m> just ↑eating a lot

22              because you know he may ↑be .hhhhh

23              [he may be ↑physically unwe:ll] >he may< have=

24   OT:        [>is he on any< medi↑cation,   ]

25   PSY:       =physical reasons for gaining ↑wei:[:ght,]

26   MAN:                                      [yea:h] he

27              ↑doesn't mention medi (0.6) [↑catio:n?]

28   OT:                                    [is he ↑on] >n- not<

29              on olanzapi:ne or anything that ↑might ↑o:f,

30   CHR:       °mm°

31   SOC :      there's ↑no:: medication on

32   CHR:       [I don't]

33   MAN:       [nothing] listed

34   SOC:       °no:: listed medic[ation°]

35   MAN:                         [ri:ght]

36              (0.4)

37   CHR:       .hhh u:::m I ↑think e::r (0.4) I think y- I think

38              >you're probably< right chris l- le:ts (0.4) book

39              in an em dee ↑tee:? ↑for ↑him?
```

This extract follows a team discussion about the risks for a particular service user. The health and social care team manager suggests that a separate MDT meeting may be required because of the complexity of his case. He introduces the idea that the service user is physically unhealthy at lines 2 and 4 and the chair shows strong agreement with this stance in line 3, with a louder and fast, 'I know'. The manager then goes on to consider the social circumstances of the service user in lines 6–10. In lines 11 and 12, the psychiatrist interjects to question whether this is in his knowledge domain given the mention of physical health (weight). He asks whether he 'should' see the service user. The question seems to respect the deontic status (and stance here) of the team in having authority to make this decision, but also ask them for permission to say that he should go, given perhaps his deontic status derived from his profession as a psychiatrist. He then gives an account for his suggestion in lines 13 and 17, but this account, and his bid for a higher deontic stance to make the decision, is dismissed by the manager in line 14, using an historical claim—'he was always physically'. The psychiatrist continues, suggesting that weight gain can be for reasons other than just weight gain. This is not taken up, and indeed, the OT then speaks in overlap with the psychiatrist on line 23 to ask about medication, which the manager responds to in line 26, rather than responding to the psychiatrist. The conversation then continues about the medication, and the psychiatrist is ignored. Here, it seems that the deontic authority of the manager (also chairing the meeting) the possible historically based epistemic stance (as opposed to professional epistemic status and stance which the psychiatrist seemed to claim), and the reactions of the other team members, seemed to lead to the psychiatrists voice being drowned out.

This exploration is brought to a close by the health and social care team manager's 'right' at line 35. The chair then returns to the earlier suggestion of having an MDT for this service user as opposed to allowing the psychiatrist the time and space to explore his concerns. The chair then continues to 'book in an MDT' for the service user, and without addressing the psychiatrist's concerns.

Challenging the Psychiatrist

In Extract 4, we see not just how the psychiatrist is ignored, but how he is directly challenged and how he challenges the expectations from him. In this example, he attempts to use his own epistemic status and stance based on his professional knowledge of the situation and how assessments are conducted. However, this is challenged by the manager claiming a deontic status, perhaps for the MDT, where the MDT is responsible for all of the list of patients, with limited resources and so how professional time is used needs careful measurement. The extract follows an extended discussion about a different service user within the same team. The GP had raised a concern about his weight, and there had followed a discussion about his poor diet and sedentary lifestyle. At this stage, the psychiatrist queried the service user's physical health. This was not taken up by the team, who moved onto discussion about social concerns. The psychiatrist then enquired whether the service user was someone he needed to see (in line 1).

Extract 4: Example of an Incongruent View of the Psychiatrist's Deontic Status

(CHR) chai, (PSY) psychiatrist (PSY), (SLT) speech and language therapist (SLT). Also present in the meeting were a minute taker, occupational therapist and physiotherapist.

```
1      PSY:  is he someone I need to ↑see::: or

2      CHR:  er, (.) >I think< it's somebody who:::: (0.6) you'd do

3            well to come to the em dee tee about (.) but I don't know

4            if there's anybody: (.) y- I don't think you need to go

5            and s- (.) rush out and see °him°.

6      PSY:  so, (0.6) cos I ↑can't, (.) have an opinion of him if I

7            don't ↑see him, °because,°

8      CHR:  °yeah well you can° ↑well, °you c'n°

9      PSY:  (°↑visit°)

10     CHR:  go and vi↑si:t, (0.4) but ↑le:t's just >I I< think it's

11           ↑worth seei::ng who else is invol̲ved it's [been an]=

12     PSY:                                             [°°(?)°°]

13     CHR:  =internal referral, (0.4) .hh hh ↑no it's come from the

14           gee pee but ↑sara::h [and jill,]

15     SLT:                       [sarah and] ji::ll (.) °are involved°

16
```

The psychiatrist's query 'is he someone I need to see or' in line 1 orientates to a shared understanding of who is appropriate for the psychiatrist to review. Simultaneously, by asking the MDT, it suggests that they have the deontic status to make decisions about who he 'ought' to see. In lines 2–5 the chair, after a short pause, responds but then repairs their response and instead invites the psychiatrist to the MDT. The hesitation and repair suggests this might be considered as a dispreferred response. This response from the chair is clear, 'I don't think you need to go and rush out and see him'—but it is also hesitant, displayed as if it might be dispreferred. The psychiatrist's response in line 6 is also dispreferred. It begins with a 'so' as if a precursor to an upshot, and then a pause. This is followed by a clear account that 'he can not have an opinion if he does not see him', which seems to invalidate the chair's position that attending the MDT alone would be helpful. The chair then states that the psychiatrist can go and visit (lines 8 and 10), but goes on to account for his hesitation, demonstrating a greater knowledge the local service practices by suggesting that others might also be involved. In this extract, there is an orientation towards the psychiatrist's obligations, but also the responsibilities of the team. The chair makes the decision regarding the appropriateness of the psychiatrist visiting the service user and so displays his deontic right to decide the most appropriate course of action.

Implications for Interprofessional Working

- Power can be positive as well as negative: acknowledging people's professional expertise is helpful.
- The MDT as a group can exert considerable influence in terms of who is allowed to speak or not allowed to speak. It might be worth reflecting on the shared understandings of the team, and how easy it is for new people to access these interactional practices.
- It might be helpful not to assume that professional hierarchies will inevitably influence team meetings—other knowledge types such as of specific professional expertise, service organisation and historical knowledge of service users can also help to increase epistemic or deontic stance within a team meeting.

Summary

Our main finding here was how deontic and epistemic stance and status can work independently of traditional hierarchical structures that have been the focus of prior research (Baker et al., 2011; Gair & Hartery, 2001; McCallin, 1999). This helps to reveal some of the complex ways in which power might operate within MDT meetings. What was often important in these excerpts was the epistemic stance derived from personal knowledge of service users, and the broader organisation of the service. These became more important than hierarchy in accounting for decisions that were made. These decisions also implied a deontic order. Some deontic authority was derived from which professional should have authority in making decisions (the manager, or the MDT as a group, for example). Our findings extend the work of Heritage (2012) by examining not just dyadic, but group interactions, where there are added considerations in terms of power, including the group responses to individuals, for example, the group responding to correct an individual, or collective ignoring of an individual's response. The analysis also demonstrated how power itself is not inherently problematic—examples were shown of how an MDT might work together by respecting the professional experience of individual members, demonstrating 'domain specific' authority.

In terms of theory, we suggest that it might be important to go beyond research that focuses on communication in health care, and to reflect on how power can be theorised in different contexts. In drawing on Pratto's (2015) relational conceptualisation of power, our example illustrates how the group (in this case the MDT) were able to control the decision-making, through together defining different forms of epistemic stance that they would respect. The degree of respect or acknowledgement in these contexts did not automatically come from the profession of the speaker, but was also affected by their epistemic stance in terms of historical or broader operational knowledge of the service. In some cases, the deontic status of the group and individuals such as the manager was also prioritised over profession. These features seem key to understanding how interprofessional working might really be engaged in a way that does not prioritise professional affiliation.

References

Anspach, R. R. (1993). *Deciding who lives: Fateful choices in the intensive-care nursery.* Berkeley: University of California Press.

Atwal, A., & Caldwell, K. (2005). Do all health and social care professionals interact equally: A study of interactions in multidisciplinary teams in the United Kingdom. *Scandinavian Journal of Caring Sciences, 19*(3), 268–273.

Baker, L., Egan-Lee, E., Martimianakis, M. A., & Reeves, S. (2011). Relationships of power: Implications for interprofessional education. *Journal of Interprofessional Care, 25*(2), 98–104.

Butler, R. R., Monsalve, M. N., Segre, A. M., Herman, T., Polgreen, P. M., Erickson, H. L., & Comellas, A. P. (2018). Estimating time physicians and other healthcare workers spend with patients in an intensive care unit using a sensor network. *American Journal of Medicine, 131*(8), 972.e9–972.e15. https://doi.org/10.1016/j.amjmed.2013.03.015.

Christofides, S., Johnstone, L., & Musa, M. (2012). 'Chipping in': Clinical psychologists' descriptions of their use of formulation in multidisciplinary team working. *Psychology and Psychotherapy, 85*(4), 424–435.

Cott, C. (1997). "We decide, you carry it out": A social network analysis of multidisciplinary long-term care teams. *Social Science and Medicine, 45*(9), 1411–1421.

Cott, C. (1998). Structure and meaning in multidisciplinary teamwork. *Sociology of Health & Illness, 20*(6), 848–873.

Crosby, B. C. (2010). Leading in the shared-power world of 2020. *Public Administration Review, 70*(s1), s69–s77.

Currie, G., & Suhomlinova, O. (2006). The impact of institutional forces upon knowledge sharing in the UK NHS: The triumph of professional power and the inconsistency of policy. *Public Administration, 84*(1), 1–30.

Currie, G., Finn, R., & Martin, G. (2010). Role transition and the interaction of relational and social identity: New nursing roles in the English NHS. *Organization Studies, 31*(7), 941–961.

Currie, G., Lockett, A., Finn, R., Martin, G., & Waring, J. (2012). Institutional work to maintain professional power: Recreating the model of medical professionalism. *Organization Studies, 33*(7), 937–962.

Dunne, F. J., Jaffar, K., & Latoo, J. (2013). Poor ways of working: Dilution of care and responsibility. *British Journal of Medical Practitioners, 6*(2), a613.

Gair, G., & Hartery, T. (2001). Medical dominance in multidisciplinary teamwork: A case study of discharge decision-making in a geriatric assessment unit. *Journal of Nursing Management, 9*(1), 3–11.

Gerstner, C. R., & Day, D. V. (1997). Meta-analytic review of leader-member exchange theory: Correlates and construct issues. *Journal of Applied Psychology, 82*, 827–844. https://doi.org/10.1037/0021-9010.82.6.827.

Haslam, S. A., Reicher, S. D., & Platow, M. J. (2011). *The new psychology of leadership*. New York: Psychology Press.

Henneman, E. A., Lee, J. L., & Cohen, J. I. (1995). Collaboration: A concept analysis. *Journal of Advanced Nursing, 21*(1), 103–109.

Heritage, J. (2010). Questioning in medicine. In A. F. Freed & S. Ehrlich (Eds.), *"Why do you ask?" The function of questions in institutional discourse* (pp. 42–68). New York, NY: Oxford University Press.

Heritage, J. (2012). Epistemics in action: Action formation and territories of knowledge. *Research on Language and Social Interaction, 45*(1), 1–29.

Heritage, J., & Raymond, G. (2012). Navigating epistemic landscapes: Acquiescence, agency and resistance in responses to polar questions. Questions: Formal, functional and interactional perspectives. In J. P. de Ruiter (Ed.), *Questions: Formal, functional and interactional perspectives* (pp. 179–192). Cambridge: Cambridge University Press.

Janss, R., Rispens, S., Segers, M., & Jehn, K. A. (2012). What is happening under the surface? Power, conflict and the performance of medical teams. *Medical Education, 46*(9), 838–849.

Johnson, S. L. (2009). International perspectives on workplace bullying among nurses: A review. *International Nursing Review, 56*(1), 34–40.

Klein, R. (1982). Performance, evaluation and the NHS: A case study in conceptual perplexity and organizational complexity. *Public Administration, 60*(4), 385–407.

Koeck, C. (2014). Imbalance of power between patients and doctors. *British Medical Journal, 349*, g7485.

Landmark, A. M. D., Gulbrandsen, P., & Svennevig, J. (2015). Whose decision? Negotiating epistemic and deontic rights in medical treatment decisions. *Journal of Pragmatics, 78*, 54–69.

Lipman, T. (2000). Power and influence in clinical effectiveness and evidence based medicine. *Family Practice, 17*(6), 557–563.

Maddock, A. (2014). Consensus or contention: An exploration of multidisciplinary team functioning in an Irish mental health context. *European Journal of Social Work, 18*(2), 246–261.

Marriott, S. (2008). *Inclusion and exclusion in the NHS: Power, innovation and rejection in nursing.* Doctoral dissertation, University of Hertfordshire.

Marshall, P., & Robson, R. (2005). Preventing and managing conflict: Vital pieces in the patient safety puzzle. *Healthcare Quarterly, 8*(Sp).

McCallin, A. (1999). *Revolution in healthcare: Altering Systems, changing behaviour.* PhD, Gaithersburg.

Nadzam, D. M. (2009). Nurses' role in communication and patient safety. *Journal of Nursing Care Quality, 24*(3), 184–188.

Oborn, E., & Dawson, S. (2010). Knowledge and practice in multidisciplinary teams: Struggle, accommodation and privilege. *Human Relations, 63*(12), 1835–1857.

Ogland-Hand, S. M., & Zeiss, A. M. (2000). Interprofessional health care teams. In V. Molinari (Ed.), *Professional psychology in long term care: A comprehensive guide* (pp. 257–277). New York, NY: Hatherleigh Press.

Pratto, F. (2015). On power and empowerment. *British Journal of Social Psychology, 55*(1–20). https://doi.org/10.1111/bjso.12135.

Propp, K. M., Apker, J., Zabava Ford, W. S., Wallace, N., Serbenski, M., & Hofmeister, N. (2010). Meeting the complex needs of the health care team: Identification of nurse—Team communication practices perceived to enhance patient outcomes. *Qualitative Health Research, 20*(1), 15–28.

Raymond, G., & Heritage, J. C. (2006). The epistemics of social relations: Owning grandchildren. *Language in Society, 35,* 677–705.

Reeves, S., Rice, K., Conn, L. G., Miller, K. L., Kenaszchuk, C., & Zwarenstein, M. (2009). Interprofessional interaction, negotiation and non-negotiation on general internal medicine wards. *Journal of Interprofessional Care, 23*(6), 633–645.

Rowlands, S., & Callen, J. (2013). A qualitative analysis of communication between members of a hospital-based multidisciplinary lung cancer team. *European Journal of Cancer Care, 22*(1), 20–31.

Stevanovic, M., & Peräkylä, A. (2012). Deontic authority in interaction: The right to announce, propose, and decide. *Research on Language and Social Interaction, 45*(3), 297–321.

Stevanovic, M., & Peräkylä, A. (2014). Three orders in the organization of human action: On the interface between knowledge, power, and emotion in interaction and social relations. *Language in Society, 43*(2), 185–207.

Turner, J. C. J. (1990). *Social influence.* Milton Keynes: Open University Press.

Weber, M., Lukes, S., & Webb, P. D. (1986). Domination by economic power and by authority. In S. Lukes (Ed.), *Power.* New York: New York University Press.

Yoon, D. J., & Bono, J. E. (2016). Hierarchical power and personality in leader-member exchange. *Journal of Managerial Psychology, 31*(7), 1198–1213. https://doi.org/10.1108/JMP-03-2015-0078.

6

'Unspoken' Outcomes: The Unintended Consequences of Interactions in MDT Meetings as Supporting Staff Well-Being and the Delivery of Compassionate Care

Lindsay Aikman

Introduction

Narratives around the importance of compassion in health care are now ubiquitous, and rightly so. The National Health Service (NHS), in the UK, is ever more aware of the need for compassion within clinical practice, as determined by the investigations of a number of scandals in recent years. However, the breadth and depth of research exploring how compassionate care is operationalised is not yet as extensive. This chapter is based on research conducted within team meetings in chronic pain care services, whose model of multidisciplinary working is well established within mental health care. It seeks to better understand the wider functions served by multidisciplinary team (MDT) meetings insofar as how they may support the cultivation of staff well-being and compassionate care. (See Chapter 2)

L. Aikman (✉)
Livewell Southwest, Plymouth, UK
e-mail: lindsay.aikman@nhs.net

© The Author(s) 2018
C. Smart and T. Auburn (eds.), *Interprofessional Care and Mental Health*,
The Language of Mental Health, https://doi.org/10.1007/978-3-319-98228-1_6

MDT meetings are resource-intensive, and understanding how they contribute to the effective running of services helps to determine whether they should be preserved and protected. Indeed although the provision of regular MDT meetings has been described as a critical component of chronic pain services, provision has been found to be highly variable (Kailainathan, Humble, Dawson, Cameron, Gokani & Lidder, 2017). Whilst MDT effectiveness studies have focused on measuring tangible meeting outcomes, including resulting changes made to treatment plans (Chinai, Bintcliffe, Armstrong, Teape, Jones & Hosie, 2013), an emphasis on measurable outputs means less attention has been paid to less tangible functions served by multidisciplinary professionals coming together in such spaces. In keeping with terms used by services in the research, MDT will be used to refer to the groups of professionals working together, and the people who access such services will be referred to as patients.

Care providers often find themselves supporting people who experience chronic and persistent difficulties, in this case relentless pain. Solutions to patients' suffering can be infrequent and the focus is on acceptance and pain management. The burden of experiencing chronic pain finds itself reflected in a wide range of countertransferential feelings for clinicians (Das, 2014). That is the feelings that arise in the clinician, in response to working with a patient. Providers of chronic pain care have described the personal toll this work takes on their well-being and have linked it to feelings of frustration, guilt and discontentment (Matthias, Parpart, Nyland, Huffman, Stubbs, Sargent, 2010). At the same time, healthcare staff are expected to continue to be able to deliver high-quality compassionate care. The principal challenge is how care providers can consistently be the best versions of themselves as clinicians, whilst negotiating demanding service contexts and emotionally charged clinical practice.

Emotional Challenges for Care Providers

It is impossible to separate great quality care from compassionate care. In thinking about what compassionate care involves, Gilbert (2014) defines compassion as broadly comprising of two processes: firstly tuning into a person's suffering and then a more action-oriented component in doing something about it. Blocks in either of these processes are likely to be problematic in the delivery of compassionate care. To visualise what this means in practical terms, imagine a clinician has been moved by someone's suffering but becomes stuck in knowing how to help them; not only will this impact the care the patient receives but this 'stuckness' can leave clinicians feeling helpless, overwhelmed or exhausted. Equally problematic is if a care provider is very busy trying to 'do' things but has lost connection with the patient's distress to guide their actions; this could be conceived as an unintentional protective strategy on the part of a stressed or exhausted worker, we might think of this as becoming burned out. The well-being of the clinician, then, is intrinsically tied to the care that they offer.

Burnout is widespread within healthcare staff (Dev, Fernando, Lim, & Consedine, 2018) and is defined by three dimensions of exhaustion, cynicism and inefficacy (Maslach, Schaufeli, & Leiter, 2001). It affects clinical work, the clinician's own well-being, and can have knock-on effects for the clinician's family and colleagues (Cocker & Joss, 2016). Compassion fatigue is a compassion-related form of burnout (Dev, Fernando, Lim, & Consedine, 2018) and is described as a common state where a person is no longer able to deal with the costs of caring (Figley, 1995). A number of factors have been suggested to protect workers from burnout, including stronger relationships among colleagues (Abu-Bader, 2000; Murray, Logan, Simmons, Kramer, Brown, Hake, 2009) and self-compassion (Dev et al., 2018). It has further been suggested that increased perception of organisational compassion predicts workers' level of compassion for others (Henshall, Alexander, Molyneux, Gardiner, & McLellan, 2018).

Research into the factors that build closer relationships suggests that creating psychological safety and trust within teams is key. These are two of the four leadership responsibilities that reinforce safe, reliable and effective health care, according to the Institute for Healthcare Improvement (Frankel, Haraden, Federico, & Lenoci-Edwards, 2017) and that predict engagement in collaborative learning to improve healthcare services (Nembhard & Edmondson, 2006).

Team psychological safety is a shared perception that the team provides a safe environment for interpersonal risk-taking (Edmondson, 1999). The way interpersonal risk-taking is responded to by a team further shapes people's perceptions of psychological safety within the team. This idea is central to effective participation in MDT meetings where the quality of the discussion relies on the willingness of individuals to allow themselves to show vulnerability in discussing their own clinical challenges as well as feeling able to speak up and offer different perspectives to colleagues.

By focusing on MDT interactions in detail, this project sought to consider the relational, restorative or supportive features of MDT meetings and, in turn, the less tangible or unspoken outcomes that they may offer.

Project Overview

Naturalistic design is crucial in Conversation Analytic research (Potter & Hepburn, 2005); here this means that the focus is on the actual talk that takes place in MDT meetings. This project involved five chronic pain services from different UK NHS Trusts. A key factor of engagement was to support research that helped articulate or evidence what MDT meetings achieve in order to protect these spaces in the face of increasing pressure and performance targets for direct clinical activity.

Ethical approval was granted through Plymouth University to audio record MDT meetings without the researcher present. Twelve meetings from five teams were audio-recorded totalling 14 hours and 42 minutes of meeting talk, with consent sought from each group member ahead of every meeting. Teams were in charge of the recording themselves, including pausing the recording at any point if it felt appropriate to do so, and two teams exercised this right. Patient identifiable data was removed from recordings prior to transcription using audio software. The multi-layered ethical issues relating to projects such as this are developed in Chapter 3.

The research revealed heterogeneity in meeting structure in terms of frequency and duration. Some services held weekly meetings, some fortnightly and some monthly, and meetings ranged from 17 minutes to 1 hour 53 minutes in length. Two types of MDT meeting emerged: clinical and business. Clinical MDT meetings were forums for discussing patient interventions and two teams adopted this format alone. Business MDT meetings addressed service-related issues which was a format followed by one team. The remaining two teams combined both approaches. Group membership also varied, with some meetings being between colleagues who more frequently work together and some involving a wider range of professionals. Whilst this study grouped all data together, further insights regarding the value, purpose and function of MDT meetings could benefit from unpicking these differences. After orthographic transcription, the author used 'unmotivated listening' to identify six initial collections relating to patterns of interaction (following Ten Have, 2007). Patterns were refined by continuing to check the corpus of data for consistency. Target sequences were identified using multiple approaches, including searching transcripts for terms such as 'MDT', analysing repeated actions, such as introducing patient information and subjectively identifying patterns such as disagreement, through specific linguistic devices. Samples from the different collections were then analysed in a more detailed Jeffersonian-transcribed format. Interactional practices were examined in relation to the functions they might serve, and refined according to the research aims. Sequences exemplifying the practices were analysed in depth by the author and discussed with the research team and a conversation analysis data group.

Results

The conventions by which people organise their contributions in meetings do not necessarily follow the conventions of talk in everyday situations (see Chapter 4). This can be connected to having structural features such as an agenda, a chairperson and a clear purpose

(Drew & Heritage, 1992; Svennevig, 2012). The meetings in the study were conducted with a sense of purpose and awareness of time; there was usually someone to chair the meeting, although this was not necessarily the team leader, and an agenda was followed. Interactions in MDT meetings occur against a backdrop of professional affiliations and this orientation to different domains of professionals' knowledge determines people having different 'rights' and 'obligations' to speak on different topics at different times; this is known as epistemic authority (Heritage, 2012). Power can also be understood as reflecting people's rights to shape future courses of action, known as deontic authority (Stevanovic & Peräkylä, 2012). Almost all clinicians contributed to MDT meeting discussions perhaps reflecting a seemingly 'flatter' hierarchy than might be observed in other settings. Whilst not exhaustive, the following analysis outlines three interactional practices that were observed in the MDT meetings: seeking help, airing frustration in clinical work and naming tensions within the team.

Seeking Help

As might be expected, staff used the MDT meeting to seek advice on their clinical work (see also Chapter 9). Advice requests could be made in different ways including overt requests, such as "I'd like to get the take of the whole team", and more implicit requests, such as saying "I don't know what to do next with this patient". This is in line with advice seeking strategies outlined by Heritage and Sefi (1992). These sequences were typically characterised by some level of 'stuckness' in the direction of the patient's care. The following extract (Extract 1) is from a discussion where an overt request for advice had already been made and opened up a discussion, with multiple colleagues making suggestions. No decision had yet been made and this is a repeat request for input.

Extract 1: Seeking Help

(Participants: PH1 = physiotherapist.1,   PH2 = physiotherapist.2, PSY = psychologist)

```
1  PH1:    you kno:w I said we:ll, (0.8) let's put

2          everything on hold physio wise until I've

3          spoken to the em dee ↑tee::, (.) but it's,

4          (0.4) >how do< we::,

5  PSY:    ↑°mm:::°

6          (0.8)

7  PH1:    help him (.) almost by not helping him go

8          round on a ↑merry go

9          [rou:nd agai:n]

10 PH2:    [we ↑also thou]ght it might be

11         helpfu::l, (.) for someone (0.4) somewhe:re

12         (0.4) .hh to spend some time (.) doing a bit

13         of (0.4) pattern (0.6) pattern recognition with

14         him (0.6) ↑that, (.) this has been going

15         [o:::n] (.) [for] ten yea[rs<

           lines 16-19 omitted

20 PH2:    >I mean< we're basically we're sayi:ng that

21         within a physio context (0.6) that ↑there

22          ↑there's (0.4) ↑not ↑much ↑more we can

23          ↑offer,How do we know this is help seeking?
```

The speaker invites input from others by asking them "how do we help him?" (Lines 4, 7) and removes themselves from being a solution by stating "there's not much more we can offer" (lines 22–23). This is presented not as we don't know what to do, but that our expertise has been exhausted. So it not only seeks help but also does face work for the physiotherapists—that they are not deficient or incompetent in some way. This practice indirectly seeks help by moving the obligation on to those with expertise in an alternative or new epistemic domain. This extract exemplifies two interesting features of seeking help: ways to increase the obligation on others to help and how to moderate the intensity of the request.

Increasing the obligation for support: Quoting from a conversation with the patient (lines 1–3) raises Physiotherapist.1's epistemic claim by bringing the patient back into the discussion, and reasserting their needs (lines 7–9). They relay that the patient is expecting this to be discussed in the MDT which moves the accountability for an outcome to the whole team; this shifts power outwards. Physiotherapist.2's use of "we also thought" (line 10) displays alignment with physiotherapist.1 and positions ownership of the request within the whole physiotherapy team, rather than one individual.

Moderating the request: Whilst creating a sense of obligation, staff also spoke in ways that lessened the intensity of the request making it seem that it is not directed at specific individuals. By referring to "the MDT" (line 3), rather than 'you', Physiotherapist.1 externalises the request to a more distant third party, as does Physiotherapist.2's use of "someone somewhere" (line 11).

Airing Frustrations in Clinical Work

Frustrations were aired when clinician(s) shared that they were finding an aspect of the clinical work challenging. It tended to be accompanied by having reached an impasse of some sort. Just prior to this sequence (see Extract 2), Doctor.1 had introduced the purpose for bringing this case to the MDT meeting as "it's not so much that I don't know what to do, but I'm surprised at how it's going" (not shown in the extract). It was unclear why the speaker chose to bring this material to the meeting; this action lacking congruence with the declaration that it is not about getting advice.

Extract 2:

(Participants: DR1 = doctor.1, DR2 = doctor.2, PSY = psychologist)

```
1    DR1: ↑yes but this >woman< is hu::gely she's very

2         a↑sser↑tive with me

3    DR2: yeah,

4    DR1: you know, (.) ↑really ↑wants ↑it ↑do::ne >an- I<

5         ↑gotta ↑have ↑it ↑do::ne and ↑why was my

6         a↑ppointment la::te?

7    DR2: .hh but did she have post natal de↑pression and it

8         [was a (?)]

9    DR1: [well I - ] my initial a↑↑sse↑↑ssment (letter) says

10        she wa:s,

11   DR2: °mm°

12   PSY: I'm just wondering abou:t (.) like maybe ↑pee ↑tee

13        ↑ess ↑↑dee::: an-, (0.4) did she have a traumatic

14        [↑bi::::rth ↓or °(?)°]

15   DR1: [well (not) really::,] you see I ↑have, (.)

16        ↓verbally ↓I ↓don't think I've mentioned it in the

17        letter (.) broached to he:::r (0.4) psychological

18        and behavioral type ↑issues and she's been ↑very

19        ↑reluctant,

     <lines 18-28 omitted>

29   DR2: [wel]l ↑I think it's [worth]

30   DR1:                      [(?)  ] (.) that's why I

31        brought her he:re (.) cos I thought that e:::r
```

How Do We Know This Is Frustration?

We can infer that Doctor.1 is about to offer a critical description of the patient, but self-repairs and downgrades it to "she's very assertive with me" (lines 1–2). Doctor.1 then relays the patient's complaint using a 3-part list (lines 4–6), which affirms a breadth or globality to it (Hutchby & Wooffitt, 2008). In the final two parts to the list, Doctor.1 voices the patient: "I gotta have it done and why was my appointment late?" Often such voicing contains an element of evaluating the stance of the person being voiced and here it indicates Doctor.1 evaluates the patient's requests or queries as impolite, assertive and unreasonable. The intonation contour and elongations further indicate frustration.

How Do Colleagues Respond to the Frustration?

Doctor.2 and the Psychologist make contributions that could develop the problem in a different way by introducing post-natal depression and PTSD to the discussion (lines 7–8 & 12–13). In so doing, the MDT self-regulated the discussion away from troubles-telling (Jefferson, 1988) and back into the clinical domain. The offering of suggestions indicates they may have receipted Doctor.1's description of the problem (lines 1–6) as describing an 'untoward state of affairs' which can be seen as a form of soliciting advice (Heritage & Sefi, 1992).

The airing of frustration was closed down by colleagues' contributions and the progressivity of the talk was not smooth thereafter, suggesting the speakers were not aligned in their goals for the conversation. Doctor.1 holds the epistemic claims to knowledge of the patient but answers vaguely in response to questions (lines 9–10, 15–18). His vagueness does not facilitate exploration of alternatives and could be viewed as resistance to advice. The advice giving may have been premature or unwanted. It could be inferred that a purpose for bringing this discussion to the MDT meeting was not to seek advice but to air frustration.

Naming Tensions Within the Team

MDT meetings also discussed service-related issues, such as recruitment, equipment issues and service development. In the following extract (Extract 3), the team had been discussing a recent move into a temporary office, for which the specialist nurse had done much of the practical arranging. Someone had just asked if the specialist nurse could get a toner cartridge for the printer in the temporary office and they had agreed. The doctor, who is also the clinical lead, challenged this.

Extract 3:

(Participants: DR = doctor, SN = specialist nurse, PSY = psychologist)

```
1   DR:   really? (.) are y- are yo[-]

2   SN:                        [y]ea:h >no n[o<]

3   DR:                                  [re]ally?

4   SN:   ye::s yeah (0.4) [°yeah (fi-)°]

5   DR:                  [d'you think] these ↑tasks are

6         going to start tailing ↑off ↑quite soon ((SN name))

7         cause,

8   SN:   >i- i-< (.) it's just something it's just, (0.4)

9         matter of picking one up and bringing it across it's

10        not a problem.

11  DR:   okay >I mean< ↑I::, (.) >okay [so<]

12  SN:                            [ye]ah

13  DR:   ↑ques↑↑tio:n? (.) should [we::] (1.0) I mean you've

14        just=

15  SN:                        [yeah]

16  DR:   =done fantas[tica]lly well and you put your hand up

17        and=
```

```
18   SN:              [yeah]

19   DR:   =said I'll °↓do ↓this° (0.4) thank you

20   SN:   mm

21   DR:   do we need to, (0.4) distribute (.) the tasks around

22         everybody else a bit ↑mo:re? (0.4) y'see I ↑think

23         (.) ↑I'd be getting a bit cheesed off ↑if ↑I was

24         you:, .hh .hhh

25   SN:   I ↑think what would be really helpful to ↓me:::

26   DR:   uh

27   SN:   is if people::: (0.6) could see::: (1.0) try to (.)

28         work out a possible solution them[se::lves,]

29   DR:                                     [for their] own

30         problems >↑yeah ↑yeah ↑yeah<

31   SN:   whe:n some of these thi:ngs (.) a:::re (.) not

32         necessarily (0.6) imminently hu::ge

33   DR:   ↑yep
```

Inviting others to express frustration: The doctor makes invitations to express frustration with increasing directness, initially inviting the specialist nurse to say no to the request quite gently, through the raised intonation and repetition of "really" (lines 1–3). The nurse does not receipt this and deflects their response back to talking about toner (lines 8–10). The doctor upgrades the enquiry to ask about distributing tasks (lines 21–22) followed by "I'd be getting a bit cheesed off if I were you" (lines 23–24). This accomplishes two tasks; it openly names that the nurse might be feeling frustrated whilst at the same time downgrading the intensity of the suggestion by locating it within (the doctor) themself rather than posing it as a direct question.

Creating psychological safety: The doctor creates psychological safety for the nurse to express dissatisfaction by prefacing it with comments on how well they have done and thanking them in front of everyone (lines 11–19). Despite the invitation, it seems problematic for the specialist nurse to report frustration, as indicated by the elongations and pauses (lines 25–32). Once the nurse starts to share what would be helpful, the doctor takes opportunities to affiliate with what they are saying. This is displayed through comments like 'yep' and 'yeah' (lines 26–33), which have an encouraging effect.

Discussion

How people talk to one another about their work signals how they are holding work-related material and the course of an MDT interaction can help move things in a more, or less, helpful direction. As careers span many years of service for the average clinician, it is useful to think beyond interactions as single units of communication and understand how they combine over time to shape individual practice and team culture. The sustainable delivery of compassionate care requires clinicians to be resilient enough to continue to tune into people's suffering and either know, or know how to find out, ways to help (Gilbert, 2014).

The first pattern of interaction identified in this study indicated that people used MDT meetings to seek help from colleagues. Sometimes colleagues were asking for direct input to the care itself, as was the case in Extract 1. The specific linguistic devices explored firstly how to increase the obligation for others to step in by reasserting the patient's needs and moving accountability to the whole team, and secondly how to moderate the intensity of such requests. It is valuable to balance the needs of the self with the needs of other colleagues when help-seeking: it is only a short-term gain if colleagues say yes to something only because they feel obliged to. Expressing the need for help or advice inherently contains an element of not-knowing, feeling stuck or acknowledging limits to professional knowledge and therefore necessitates interpersonal risk-taking. This is recognised by the tentative moderating of a request and the face-saving aspect to the talk (Extract 1), as well as knowing it intuitively. So, whilst people can hone their practice in terms of skilful help-seeking, it is the way that requests for help are receipted and responded to by others that determine whether the exchange ultimately proves to be beneficial. This is because responses to help-seeking shape the perception of psychological safety within the team; either fostering a trusting environment where people can openly name issues and seek opinions, or creating one where being guarded about acknowledging limitations feels necessary.

Raising awareness of how we respond to help-seeking from others therefore points towards ways we can contribute to effective team cultures. Greater responsibility for creating psychological safety resides with senior staff members, as they have more psychological safety to begin with by virtue of their positioning in the professional hierarchy (Nembhard & Edmondson, 2006). The second pattern of interaction identified in this study was the airing of frustration in clinical work. When frustration found expression it was rarely introduced as such, but rather was observed as a by-product of describing a problematic feature in the work. Extract 2 exemplified interactional features that may help us more readily identify that frustration is present, such as intonation contours, elongation and how the patient is voiced. Beyond identification, it is important to then address frustration to inform clinical practice rather than shying away from it. Acknowledging its presence can serve the function of raising the clinician's awareness of their own emotional responses and with increased awareness, they are enabled to self-regulate. It also opens up possibility for teams to exercise their responsibility in highlighting when clinicians' reactions may be inappropriately affecting their practice.

This speaks to the complexities of understanding 'collaboration' in MDTs. In Extract 2, colleagues are not 'collaborating' with Doctor.1 on the face of it, rather they are guiding the conversation to a different, and possibly more appropriate, focus. Receiving validation and support may assist colleagues in processing difficult emotions in relation to challenging work. Within the literature on compassion in health care (Mannion, 2014) and compassion fatigue (Figley, 1995), it is possible to frame how processing emotional responses can be valuable in healthcare work by lessening the burden on the clinician, thereby positively impacting their well-being and supporting the professional to engage more authentically and compassionately. Irrespective of whether a professional is responding to a sense of clinical 'stuckness' with the work, whether they are internalising some of the patient's frustrations or whether their restorative needs are more personal in nature, these interactions build transparency and trust when supportive and affiliative. However, if discussed in an environment that does not feel psychologically safe, the risk is it builds a culture of blame, criticism and fear.

The management of tensions within teams, as demonstrated in Extract 3, is hard to diarise or plan for. Issues in team dynamics may present themselves via discussion on unrelated topics and as 'live' phenomena need to be named and negotiated at that time. Extract 3 is a good example of how quickly tension can build, be acknowledged and smoothed, in this case all in less than 90 seconds. The team leader in Extract 3 used the rights associated with their position as chair to good effect and, by a process of affiliating and permission giving, enabled a potentially problematic dynamic to be validated and diffused. To some extent, this shows us how we can negotiate different emotions within the room. Regular and proactive leadership of this kind is likely to build a greater sense of affiliation and safety and conveys compassion from the organisation which in turn predicts compassion for others (Henshall, Alexander, Molyneux, Gardiner & McLellan, 2018). It is important for teams to learn how to negotiate clinical disagreement respectfully to expand perspectives. A degree of interpersonal strain in MDT meetings already likely exists owing to the creative tensions that reside between professionals trained in different disciplines (Peck & Norman, 1999; cited in Mental Health Commission, 2006). Within any team, it is not realistic to expect an absence of disagreement, so the goal might be to proactively acknowledge and manage it.

These findings connect to staff well-being and delivering compassionate care in a number of ways. They have the potential to foster better working relationships with colleagues and has this been found to protect workers from burnout (Abu-Bader, 2000; Murray et al., 2009). Over time, these interactional practices convey "how we do things around here" and such messages shape organisational culture (Manley, 2008). There is some evidence to suggest that organisational culture may influence performance in health care (Scott, Mannion, Marshall, & Davies, 2003). They also influence perception of psychological safety which reinforces safe, reliable and effective health care (Frankel et al.,

2017) and determines the degree to which clinicians are willing to take interpersonal risks in MDT meetings. This is likely to affect the depth of the MDT conversations as well as the extent to which practitioners experience these spaces as restorative. There is the opportunity for MDT meeting interactions to influence whether or not individuals come to identify with the team and this is important because identifying with one's team increases overall job satisfaction (Onyett, Pillinger, & Muijen, 1997).

Should MDT meeting experiences contribute to clinicians perceiving greater organisational compassion, this predicts greater capacity to give compassion to others (Henshall et al., 2018). We might extrapolate, therefore, that MDT meetings can offer potential benefits in terms of improving the quality of communication between professionals, offering restorative spaces for clinicians to become more aware of, and process, their emotions in relation to work and impact on the quality of compassionate care offered over time. Limitations of this project were that the analysis has been conducted on audio rather than video material; non-verbal and other contextual information was therefore not included in the analysis.

The identification of interactional practices was not exhaustive and contains subjectivity. This was moderated by having other people review extracts including peer and supervisor data sessions and participation at a Conversation Analysis data group as well as bracketing interviews whereby the researcher is interviewed to reveal issues of personal bias that may otherwise affect the research. When considering how normative the findings are of pain teams, it may also be useful to consider the impact of the 'flatter' hierarchies observed in these pain services, on the transferability of the findings to other settings. Features of chronic pain services that may contribute to this are, that clinicians in such teams are considered specialists which may alter traditional hierarchical power bases; the biopsychosocial model they operate from facilitates thoughtful consideration from all perspectives; and that these clinicians often work closely together in relatively small services which impacts upon the team dynamics.

Recommendations for interprofessional team working

- A number of interactional practices were identified in this study (seeking help, airing frustration in clinical work and naming tensions within teams). Think about these in relation to your own participation in MDT meetings.
- When seeking help, consider restating a request to reorient the MDT meeting discussion, the ways you might increase the obligation on others to help and moderate your request to reduce the risk of triggering defensive reactions from others.
- When there is resistance to advice being given, it may be useful to explore what input is being sought from the MDT. Rather than seeking literal advice, your colleague might be seeking an opportunity to process their own emotional responses in order to move forward with the work.
- Frustration is a valuable indicator of a colleague's experience.
- The care plan may or may not change as a result of an MDT discussion but staff members feeling supported, validated and less stuck cultivates clinical hopefulness and this has been shown to positively impact the therapeutic relationship with patients.
- Encourage colleagues to proactively name and manage tensions arising within the team. Being validating of others and affiliating with them is effective.
- Building trust and psychological safety within the team has been found to reinforce safe, reliable and effective health care (Frankel et al., 2017).
- If you are a senior staff member, be mindful that your position affords you greater psychological safety than other colleagues may be experiencing.
- Being aware of the unspoken functions of MDT meetings enables us to link the value of these spaces to other organisational drivers such as staff support and cultivating compassion within the organisation. Use these to encourage service providers to think more broadly about their function.

Summary

Research into MDT meetings often focuses on their direct impact on patient care. In this project, we found a range of interactional practices that flesh out some of the less tangible benefits that may contribute to the delivery of compassionate care. They have the potential to serve restorative functions for clinicians; build work cultures that promote interpersonal risk-taking and psychological safety; help teams function better and cultivate factors known to reduce burnout. The intangible qualities of some of these practices render them hard to quantify and difficult to build into a meaningful health economic argument. The way interactions are managed in MDT meetings sends messages about how team working is done. Such 'messages' can shape organisational culture (Manley, 2008) and in this way, MDT meetings should be considered mechanisms for fostering effective interprofessional working practices in health care. Being able to describe the breadth of potential benefits helps articulate why these MDT spaces are important.

Tips for doing research

- Be thoughtful about how to respect patient confidentiality in research projects such as these and address inadvertent exposure to patient identifiable data. Chapter 3 considers ethical dilemmas of these projects in more depth
- Be transparent about your ethical obligations
- Identify key structural differences in MDT meeting practices if engaging multiple teams. Be thoughtful about the impact these may have on your research
- The process of unmotivated listening can feel overwhelming in the face of large volumes of data. Be mindful of how much data you collect or tighten the focus of what you are listening out for to manage this
- Incorporate processes to minimise the impact of researcher bias in your project

---

Acknowledgements I would like to thank the five teams that took part in this project. I appreciate their willingness to allow researchers to be party to the way they conduct their work.

I would particularly like to thank each of psychologists in the team who acted as points of liaison for their respective teams.

Thanks go to my supervisors: Cordet Smart for attention to detail and unerring enthusiasm throughout the project; and Sarah Baldrey for her central role in facilitating introductions with chronic pain care teams.

I was fortunate to be part of a Conversation Analysis Research Group based at the University of Plymouth. Thank you to them for the steady flow of critical thinking and fresh perspectives on data. With special thanks to Nicole Parish, my colleague, friend and fellow CA researcher, for her endless ability to inspire and find ways we can share our research with the world.

Most of all I would like to thank my partner, Chris, for his support and being the voice in my head encouraging my own self-care.

References

Abu-Bader, S. H. (2000). Work satisfaction, burnout, and turnover among social workers in Israel: A causal diagram. *International Journal of Social Welfare, 9,* 191–200.

Chinai, N., Bintcliffe, F., Armstrong, E., Teape, J., Jones, B., & Hosie, K. (2013). Does every patient need to be discussed at a multidisciplinary team meeting? *Clinical radiology, 68*(8), 780–784.

Cocker, F., & Joss, N. (2016). Compassion fatigue among healthcare, emergency and community service workers: A systematic review. *International Journal of Environmental Research and Public Health, 13*(6), 618.

Das, M. (2014). CAT and the mind-body conundrum of chronic pain. *Reformulation* (Summer), 29–32.

Dev, V., Fernando, A. T., Lim, A. G., & Consedine, N. S. (2018). Does self-compassion mitigate the relationship between burnout and barriers to compassion? A cross-sectional quantitative study of 799 nurses. *International Journal of Nursing Studies, 81,* 81–88.

Drew, P., & Heritage, J. (1992). *Talk at work: Interaction in institutional settings.* Cambridge: Cambridge Univeristy Press.

Edmondson, A. (1999). Psychological safety and learning behavior in work teams. *Administrative Science Quarterly, 44*(2), 350–383.

Figley, C. R. (1995). Compassion fatigue: Toward a new understanding of the costs of caring. In B. H. Stamm (Ed.), *Secondary traumatic stress: Self-care issues for clinicians, researchers, and educators* (pp. 3–28). Baltimore, MD: The Sidran Press.

Frankel, A., Haraden, C., Federico, F., & Lenoci-Edwards, J. (2017). *A framework for safe, reliable, and effective care.* White paper. Cambridge, MA: Institute for Healthcare Improvement and Safe & Reliable Healthcare.

Gilbert, P. (2014). The origins and nature of compassion focused therapy. *British Journal of Clinical Psychology, 53*(1), 6–41.

Henshall, L. E., Alexander, T., Molyneux, P., Gardiner, E., & McLellan, A. (2018). The relationship between perceived organisational threat and compassion for others: Implications for the NHS. *Clinical Psychology & Psychotherapy, 25*(2), 231–249.

Heritage, J. (2012). The epistemic engine: Sequence organization and territories of knowledge. *Research on Language & Social Interaction, 45*(1), 30–52.

Heritage, J., & Sefi, S. (1992). Dilemmas of advice: Aspects of the delivery and reception of advice in interactions between health visitors and first-time mothers. In P. Drew & J. Heritage (Eds.), *Talk at work: Interaction in institutional settings.* Cambridge: Cambridge Univeristy Press.

Hutchby, I., & Wooffitt, R. (2008). *Conversation analysis* (2nd ed.). Cambridge: Polity Press.

Jefferson, G. (1988). On the sequential organization of troubles-talk in ordinary conversation. *Social Problems, 35*(4), 418–441.

Kailainathan, P., Humble, S., Dawson, H., Cameron, F., Gokani, S., & Lidder, G. (2017). A national survey of pain clinics within the United Kingdom and Ireland focusing on the multidisciplinary team and the incorporation of the extended nursing role. *British Journal of Pain, 12*(1), 47–57.

Manley, K. (2008). 'The way things are done around here'—Developing a culture of effectiveness: A pre-requisite to individual and team effectiveness in critical care. *Australian Critical Care, 21*(2), 83–85.

Mannion, R. (2014). Enabling compassionate healthcare: Perils, prospects and perspectives. *International Journal of Health Policy and Management, 2*(3), 115.

Maslach, C., Schaufeli, W. B., & Leiter, M. P. (2001). Job burnout. *Annual Review of Psychology, 52*(1), 397–422.

Matthias, M. S., Parpart, A. L., Nyland, K. A., Huffman, M. A., Stubbs, D. L., Sargent, C., & Bair, M. J. (2010). The patient–provider relationship in chronic pain care: Providers' perspectives. *Pain Medicine, 11*(11), 1688–1697.

Mental Health Commission. (2006). *Multidisciplinary team working: From theory to practice.* Dublin: Mental Health Commission.

Murray, M., Logan, T., Simmons, K., Kramer, M. B., Brown, E., Hake, S., & Madsen, M. (2009). Secondary traumatic stress, burnout, compassion fatigue and compassion satisfaction in trauma nurses. *American Journal of Critical Care, 18*(3), e1–e17.

Nembhard, I. M., & Edmondson, A. C. (2006). Making it safe: The effects of leader inclusiveness and professional status on psychological safety and improvement efforts in health care teams. *Journal of Organizational Behavior, 27*(7), 941–966.

Onyett, S., Pillinger, T., & Muijen, M. (1997). Job satisfaction and burnout among members of community mental health teams. *Journal of Mental Health, 6*(1), 55–66.

Potter, J., & Hepburn, A. (2005). Qualitative interviews in psychology: Problems and possibilities. *Qualitative research in Psychology, 2*(4), 281–307.

Scott, T., Mannion, R., Marshall, M., & Davies, H. (2003). Does organisational culture influence health care performance? A review of the evidence. *Journal of Health Services Research & Policy, 8*(2), 105–117.

Stevanovic, M., & Peräkylä, A. (2012). Deontic authority in interaction: The right to announce, propose, and decide. *Research on Language & Social Interaction, 45*(3), 297–321.

Svennevig, J. (2012). Interaction in workplace meetings. *Discourse Studies, 14*(1), 3–10.

Ten Have, P. (2007). *Doing conversation analysis: A practical guide.* London: Sage.

Part III

Clinical Applications—Team Formulations in Mental Health MDTs

7

Conversation Analysis of Psychological Formulation Discussions in Adult Learning Disabilities Teams

Katherine Peckitt and Cordet Smart

Introduction

This project was a conversation analytic (CA) investigation of the interaction between clinical psychologists and their colleagues in team meeting settings with a specific focus on the processes involved in team formulation discussions. The clinical psychologist's role in team settings can include facilitating discussions and reflections about the factors contributing to people's emotional distress beyond diagnostic categories. A way in which this might be conducted is through the development of joint psychological formulations in team meetings (see also Chapter 1). These might draw from a wide range of theoretical approaches in order to create a working hypothesis or a 'best guess' about the reasons for a person's difficulties (Johnstone & Dallos, 2014). The emphasis on a

K. Peckitt (✉) · C. Smart
School of Psychology, University of Plymouth, Plymouth, UK
e-mail: katherine.peckitt@tst.nhs.uk

C. Smart
e-mail: cordet.smart@plymouth.ac.uk

© The Author(s) 2018
C. Smart and T. Auburn (eds.), *Interprofessional Care and Mental Health,*
The Language of Mental Health, https://doi.org/10.1007/978-3-319-98228-1_7

formulation-based approach is to move away from the medical model and humanise the experiences of people in emotional distress. This project focused on how team members engaged with each other in the process of producing formulations during team meetings in services for adults with learning disabilities.

Existing research is primarily concerned with meetings that are explicitly devoted to psychological formulations. In contrast, this research examined the process of formulating in a range of team meetings where psychologists 'chip in' (cf. Christofides, Johnstone, & Musa, 2012). Christofides et al. (2012) suggested that rather than claim any form of entitlement or declare a summary of a patient's needs, the psychologists role is to 'chip in' or to suggest psychological directions within the discussion in wider MDT meetings. This therefore seemed an appropriate starting point to identify formulations in non-formulation meetings. The method used for the investigation of the processual nature of team formulation is conversation analysis. Conversation analysis of team formulation discussion might add to our understanding of the interactional processes between professionals, where clinical psychologists formulate 'informally' in team meetings. The objective was to identify and illustrate examples of informal team formulation to help demystify this concept.

Formulation

Formulation is a defining competency of the profession of clinical psychology (Division of Clinical Psychology, 2010) and 'is continuing to attract a great deal of attention' (Johnstone & Dallos, 2014). The aim of formulations is to inform psychological interventions, develop an understanding of service users' core problems, how they relate to social contexts and relationships with other people (Johnstone & Dallos, 2014). Formulations utilise psychological concepts and research evidence, which offer a range of explanations for how persons come to have these problems at this time in their life, including triggers and maintaining factors. Formulations can be revised in the light of new information. However, 'there are still wide variations in the conceptualisation of formulations and the empirical basis of them remains to be firmly established' (Johnstone & Dallos, 2014). Psychological formulations can either be understood as a specific event (e.g. a written letter outlining the psychological formulations) or a process (e.g. the ongoing discussion between the therapist and service user, who co-create ideas about psychological health).

Team Formulation

Team formulation draws on similar concepts to individual formulation, but aims to integrate all MDT members in order to develop joint hypotheses about service users (Hollingworth & Johnstone, 2014). The difference is that the service users are no longer the exclusive centre of attention. Instead, the focus is also on the interactive process of psychologists with other staff. In other words there is a certain shift away from service users on to staff. Research has pointed out the advantages of team formulations in clinical psychology. Staff report feeling appreciated and validated in their work (Unadkat, Quinn, Jones, & Casares, 2015) through the process of formulating together. Staff report that having protected time to discuss the complexities of work in mental health settings, as well as space to think creatively, helps gain alternative perspectives (Hollingworth & Johnstone, 2014). Staff views are that discussions increase their understanding of service users' mental health problems (Berry, Barrowclough, & Wearden, 2009; Unadkat et al., 2015) and develop better intervention planning (Hollingworth & Johnstone, 2014; Summers, 2006). Staff from a range of professions considered team formulations to improve staff and service user experiences through development of less blaming perceptions of and increased empathy for service users (Summers, 2006; Berry et al., 2016).

While the value of team formulation for both service user and staff is well established, there is less agreement on how they should be done. Christofides et al. (2012) and Hood, Johnstone, and Christofides (2013) suggest that there are different methods of 'doing team formulation', either in meetings specifically dedicated to team formulation (Berry et al., 2009; Berry et al., 2016) or informal settings, where team members formulate in conversations, team meetings or supervision. It has in fact been stressed that clinical psychologists are more likely to formulate 'informally' by 'chipping in' (Christofides et al., 2012). Psychologists report difficulties in defining the term 'team formulation' and are avoidant of using jargon terms such as 'formulation' within the meetings.

The most favourable settings for team formulation discussions have been partly discussed in the literature but there is no research to date on the interactional processes between psychologists and members of MDTs when developing team formulations. Little has been published on the process of psychologists 'informally' formulating ideas and what such interactions might look like. Subsequently, CA, a research method looking more closely at the interactive processes between people in naturally occurring conversation, was used to research these discussions in team meetings.

Conversation Analysis and Formulation

Conversation analysis makes use of naturalistic data, and therefore, the present research analysed audio-recordings to capture everyday clinical practice 'in action'. This approach examines the 'organisation of talk' (Heritage, 1984) and offers a suitable methodology for examining social actions through analysis the organisation of sequences of talk within institutional settings (Heritage & Clayman, 2010) (see Chapter 2).

Previous CA research has identified specific conversational objects as formulations (Heritage & Watson, 1979). Formulation is where one speaker summarises the talk up to that point. There are normally two types of formulation, gist, which gives the sense of the talk to that point, or upshot, which draws out some inference from the prior talk. Formulations are usually marked as such, often by prefacing the formulation with the discourse marker, 'so' and have a preference for agreement with the formulation in the responsive turn. Formulations are most frequent in institutional talk, being relatively rare in informal conversation. They are often used by news interviewers, for example for drawing out a newsworthy point from the extended talk of the interviewee. Characteristic of formulations is that they select, delete and/or transform elements of the prior talk.

In their examination of individual psychotherapy sessions, Antaki, Barnes and Leudar (2005) found that formulation serves as a way of moving the conversation into the therapists' preferred direction of talk and as an interactional way to bring about change or new understanding for the service user. Bercelli, Rossano and Viaro (2008) have extended formulation to include 'reinterpretations'. They reported that therapists can either (a) deal with the interpretations as 'something that was implicitly meant by the service user, so claiming they are still offering candidate reading of the perspective expressed by the service user; or (b) alternatively, as something that, though grounded in what the service user said, is caught and expressed from the therapist's own perspective- therefore something possibly different, and ostensibly so, from what the service user meant'. CA research therefore is helpful in identifying certain interactional features of formulation in institutional talk and our starting point was to apply some of these findings to MDT settings, where the psychologist offers a candidate psychological hypothesis to their colleagues.

Project Overview

Aim

The aim of this project was to add to the growing research on team formulation with the focus on the interactional processes between professionals, using data where clinical psychologists formulate 'informally' (Christofides et al., 2012) in a range of MDT settings.

Objectives

1. The first objective was to identify formulations that psychologists introduce 'informally' or by 'chipping in' in team settings.
2. The second objective was to illustrate different examples of formulations, in an attempt to understand the interactional organisation of this practice better.

Design

This project had a qualitative research design using naturalistic data (Tileaga & Stokoe, 2015) from clinical team discussions and CA as the methodological approach. MDT meetings were audio-recorded, transcribed orthographically and then micro-analysed using CA principles.

Participants

General MDT meetings with a focus on the process of 'chipping in' formulation ideas and the subsequent discussion formed the main data source for this project. The *MDTsInAction* data corpus consisted of business, referral, allocations, peer review and professional meetings in different service settings, including autism-specialist, pain management, dementia and adult learning disabilities services between 2015 and 2017 in the UK National Health Service.

This study selected 8 meetings (a total of 9 hours audio-recording) in adult learning disabilities services across different trusts. These meetings had the potential to provide a number of formulation discussions. People receiving LD services often present with complex physical, developmental and mental health comorbidities and good practice suggests the use of sophisticated biopsychosocial formulations to develop an understanding of the service user (Ingham & Clarke, 2009).

Professions in this project were clinical psychologists, trainee clinical psychologists, community nurses, assistant practitioners, primary care liaison nurses, senior nurse practitioners, IAPT nurses, continuing healthcare nurses, student nurses, occupational therapists, community nurse leads and administrators.

Research Process

The second challenge of the research was the identification of formulation 'talk', as it was never specifically referred to as 'psychological formulation'. Although the literature offers definitions of psychological formulations from different theoretical approaches (Dallos & Johnstone, 2014), there are few examples on how these interactions may look like when they take place between psychologists and other team members.

Think point

 The word 'psychological formulation' is not commonly used in everyday language. Consequently, how can we 'find it' in conversation?

Through conversations with clinical psychologists, the researchers derived a list of characteristics of formulation 'talk', which guided the process of identifying psychological formulation in team meetings. The list included words and phrases referencing psychological theories (e.g. CBT, attachment, trauma, schema, psychodynamic and systemic) or psychological language (e.g. anxiety, emotional, distressing, avoidant and defences) or hypotheses introduced with phrases such as 'I wonder how the XYZ felt about XYZ' or 'reflecting on your comments, I would say that XYZ'. Following this list, the recordings were explored by 'what was said, when it was said and how it was said' (Pillet-Shore, 2010). The initial extracts were also scrutinised in research meetings with specialist CA researchers. However, these discussions added to the dilemma of identifying formulation talk, as the initial examples did not seem to link with some of the characteristics as mentioned above. In fact, the audio-recordings suggested that in the majority of the MDT meetings, psychologists did not seem to be 'chipping in' formulation ideas or psychological hypothesising.

However, in meetings dedicated to one service user, sixteen occasions were identified when psychologists used psychological terminology (a peer review and professionals meeting). The commonality of these meetings was that only one service user was discussed rather than multiple service users (as in referral and allocations meetings).

Psychological Formulations: Tentative Statements with 'aha' Moments

Four episodes of a psychologist offering psychological formulations were noted in a peer review meeting. To detail, the whole formulation process would be too lengthy, but it is possible here to illustrate some of the activities as they unfold and demonstrate some of the design features of the interactions, see Extract 1.

The context of this formulation was that the 'presenter' of this service user to the team introduced the person with 'a learning disability, autistic spectrum disorder, heightened sensory needs and obsessive-compulsive disorder'. A chronology of events (including domestic violence and use of substances in the family home), presenting problems (e.g. aggressive behaviours and masturbation in public) and current interventions were listed.

Extract 1: Peer Review Meeting

G: Senior Nurse, M: Clinical Psychologist, C: Assistant Practitioner

```
1   G      ok, so so that's a little bit more clarity.

2          Does anybody got any have uhm da nalysis↑

3   M      I guess I'm just struck that ((clearing

4          throat)) >you know< victims↑ of domestic violence

5          are also those (.) children who've seen it haven't

6          they and not been kept (.) safe they are <emotional

7          victims> of domestic violence which I think is a

8          (( )) MASSIVE trauma for .hh for kids BUT uhm (.)

9          I am quite↑ intrigued by the fact that you say the

10         boys(.)the boys↑ (.) <blamed> mum for kind of

11         ALLO::WING the (.1) abuse↓ and she's she's a uh (.)

12         uhm (.) target for from Mark (.) from Mark (.)
```

```
13              isn't she and that's quite interesting interesting
14              [for ]=
15  C           [Yeah] OH ↑YEAH↓
16  M           =understanding that coz that's ye ye you don't (.)
17              know anymore at this point but (.) presumably but
18              in what sense=
19  C           some parallels there isn't there
20  M           =blame her
21  C           Yeah
22  ?           °°yeah°
23              (4)
24  M           and yes that's, yes, just not known isn't but(.)
25              interesting
26  C           It is difficult, isn't it (.)  Just because she is
27              looking after his dog and this is all I am basing
28              this on really
```

Initiating the Turn

The psychologist introduces the turn with 'I guess I am struck' (line 3), which was a recurrent feature in the design of these formulations. Through this utterance, the psychologist gains some independence of the account of the previous speaker (Bercelli et al., 2008), as it can only relate to the psychologists' position. 'I am struck' or 'I wonder' marks the introduction of a reinterpretation (Bercelli et al., 2008) through which the 'therapists forward their own perspective on an event and therefore supposedly shift the service user's [in this case the MDT member's] version of events'.

Developing the Formulation

Lines 3–8, the psychologist introduces a particular perspective on children as victims of domestic violence. There is a gradual build-up of the case, where initially the idea is mentioned that 'victims of domestic violence are also those children who've seen it […] and is a massive trauma for kids' in lines 3–8. This is a generalised statement that could be understood as a candidate source for a psychological hypothesis about this service user's experiences. Referring to domestic violence as 'it' (line 5) supports the notion of a specific understanding of domestic violence, as there is no further exploration of what it could entail. There is then a shift from the general claim to the experiences of 'the boys' [the service user and his brothers], which therefore makes this hypothesis more specific to the service user (Bolden & Angell, 2017). It is at this point that the psychologist links this claim to the account of the previous speaker by saying 'that you say' (line 9). This is a recurrent conversational feature in formulations to ground claims in the information provided by the previous speaker, as has been noted in research on formulation in individual therapy (Antaki et al., 2005). This provides evidence for the claim and works towards affiliation between the speaker and the recipient of the formulation. Also evident in this extract is the selection of details of the prior service user history, and the transformative work undertaken by the psychologist to account for this case using psychological terminology and concepts.

Response by MDT Member

The normative response for a formulation is agreement (Heritage & Watson, 1979), and in this interaction the MDT member responds with, '[Yeah] OH ↑YEAH↓' (line 15). 'Yeah' represents a news acknowledgement token and the 'OH ↑YEAH↓' is an upgrade of this acknowledgement. The rising and lowering pitch as well as the repetition of 'yeah' after 'Oh' conveys a sense of excitement and does not refer to the difficult experiences of the children, but to the excitement of a new understanding of the service users' situation. This 'change in stake token' (Heritage, 1984) can be understood as the successful establishment of a connection, and consequently it might be tentatively concluded that this formulation has achieved its aim, i.e. to develop a different understanding of the service users' difficulties (Johnstone, 2014).

Closing

After a pause of 4 seconds (line 23) and no extensions by other members of the MDT, the psychologist extends the utterance with 'and yes that's, yes, just not known isn't but(.) interesting'(lines 24–25). The psychologist refers to 'just not known' and this was a recurrent feature in formulation conversations, where members of the MDT refer to aspects of the service user as unknown to them, but also something that might be of significance to the sense-making process ('but interesting'). The psychologist is curious about an aspect that needs to be better understood. Curiosity statements are mechanisms for inviting the listeners to think along with the speaker, but can also be understood as an exploration of understanding. This reference to unknown facts about the service user's experiences is especially important when considering that the access to the service user's experiences is crucial to the process of facilitating change in therapeutic interaction (Fitzgerald, 2013). In line 26, the other clinician acknowledges this complexity of not knowing, 'it is difficult, isn't it', and then returns to a previously mentioned point, unrelated to the issue of domestic violence.

Extract 1 is an example of how the psychologist introduces a psychological concept to the discussion in a way that signifies their own position, while also grounding the hypothesis in general psychological concepts and accounts by previous speakers, a design similar to those seen in individual therapy (Bercelli et al., 2008). Another feature is the reference to the unknown complexities and potentially important aspects of people's lives. What the extract illustrates here is that the formulation brings in tentatively a psychological concept, which is taken up by a MDT member and effects some change in her understanding about the service user.

The next section discusses a different type of formulation design to illustrate variations in formulations in team meetings.

Psychological Formulations: An Opportunity to Express Emotional and Delicate Views

The analysis of a different professional meeting found that clinical psychologists brought in psychological formulations into the MDT discussion when MDT members expressed contentious views on service users. Ten short formulations were noted that specifically related to this process. Prior to these formulations, there had been sixteen occasions on which the service user's mother had been framed as difficult, either by misconstruing information, being overly involved in the care of her adult daughter, or by undermining the daughter's choices. Extract 2 is an example of an interactional design that attempts a development of a set of different formulations about the mother.

Extract 2: Professionals' Meeting (19.50-21.17: 1.4.5.04.05.2016)

H: Clinical Psychologist; P: Clinical Psychologist; M: Student Learning Disability Nurse; G: Community Nurse; S: service user under discussion

1	H	So would it be helpful to people↓ to hear what
2		our next roles will be
3	?	Yea::h
4	M	Hmm
5	H	So I guess Deb and I have deliberately (.)
6		<u>NOT</u> (.)had any involvement with S. we are
7		trying to be separate so that we are kind of
8		(.) a bit outside that and I think that the aim
9		would be
10	?	yes very separate
11	H	and yes you are right (.) about what would (.)
12		what S wants and what S's needs are (.)
13		<u>but</u> the best (.) we also <u>need</u> to think about
14		how we can help Mum in the process so that
15		she gives S more permission to do that
16		because if she (.) is (.) uhm (.) not (.) part
17		of the pro<u>cess</u>: there's more risk she will
18		<u>sabotage</u> it. Isn't it↓ So so I guess that's
19		where (.) we've been (.) kind of coming in
20	P	so that=
21	?	yeah
22	P	=is sort of supporting mum to accept

```
23              cha::nîge and (.) adapt

24    H         yep (.)=

25    ?         absolutely

26    H         =AAAND also I think to (.2) help (.)

27              feel that her voice is <heard> =

28    P         yes:

29    ?         absolutely yeah

30    H         =in IT (.) so that she can feel less powerf(.)=

31    P         yes

32    H         =less powerless

33    ?         Yes

34    H         =it in it so in a (.) but in a mo:re

35              <helpful way> I guess

36    P         yes

37    G         she is very good (.) she's very uh, pff££,

38              I know we are recording but she she could

39              actually receive an Oscar (.) because she can

40              switch her emotions (.) immediately and=

41    P         right

42    G         because on several occasions we've been at

43              Cromwell home with her

      ((8 lines omitted))

52    G         so she can present that way but that was at the

53              beginning so again, I am, I am, just saying that to

54    P         so when in a high level of stress and anxiety
```

```
55          she might

56   G      yes, yes, and I am being very conscious of

57          bringing that forward because obviously Braxton

58          is going to be taking that over
```

Initiating the Turn

The clinical psychologist (H) initiates a claim to the floor for a longer turn with a focusing question (lines 1–2: 'so would it be helpful to people to hear what our next roles will be'). This influenced the trajectory of the conversation towards the line of argument the psychologists are about to make, and it seeks the participation of the other MDT members. This initiating move is answered with acknowledgement tokens, 'yea::h' (line 3), 'hm' (line 4), which gives the go-ahead for the psychologist (H) to continue with a longer turn.

Developing the Formulation

In this example, the psychologist (H) takes the floor for an extended turn and uses this turn to develop a psychological formulation of the issues the service user (S) is experiencing especially in relation to S's mother. In lines 5–9, psychologist H starts to outline the non-involvement with the service user, justifying her position by stating that this was purposely decided and was an informed decision: 'So I guess Deb and I have deliberately (.) NOT (.) had any involvement with S.' and this is a part of the build-up towards the upcoming formulations. Before this happens, there is an acknowledgement of a potential objection 'and yes you are right' (line 11), where she addresses the MDT member M, who is promoting service user S's interests and is the strongest voice about the 'difficult mother'. Psychologist H acknowledges M's position and then extends her turn with 'but the best (.)' (line 13). This is a direct challenge as seen in the 'but' but even more so by using 'the best'. She stops at this point and repairs by softening with the explanation of the 'need to help mum' (line 14).

The formulation process about the mother continues in lines 16–18. Stating that 'if she [the mother] (.) is (.) uhm (.) not (.) part of the pro-cess: there's more risk she will <u>sabotage</u> it'. The pauses in between words (.) indicate a certain delicacy about this topic and that the psychologist is hesitant in formulating her sentence. It can also be read as a sign that the involvement with the mother is 'risky' or difficult and that the mother could be interruptive ('sabotage').

Here, psychologist P joins the process and produces a recognisable formulation as a conversation object. It is marked as an upshot summary of the account provided by the clinical psychologist (H): 'so that is sort of supporting mum to accept cha::n↑ge and (.) adapt' (lines 20, 22–23). This reframing (Brocelli et al., 2008) of the initial account displays the canonical features of conversational formulation by selecting elements of the prior talk, deleting others and here in particular transforming the prior talk. This transformation is designed to mitigate a potential reading of H's account as overly harsh and provide an explicit positive reading of the course of action described by H. Another team member responds with a high-grade agreement with this formulation ('absolutely', line 25).

Psychologist H then extends her account of their course of action concerning the mother in lines 26/7, 30/32, and 34/35, which refer to her being 'heard', her feelings of 'powerless'-ness and being more 'helpful'. The extensions of the formulations about the mother are retrospectively an affiliation with the upshot formulation provided by the Psychologist P and prospectively a build-up towards her goal of gaining the acceptance of the other MDT members (cf. Bolden & Angell, 2017).

Response by MDT Member

Lines 37–40 show the clinician G pursuing the oppositional line of argument that the mother is purposefully being difficult and refers to her behaviours as an act. 'She is very good (.) she's very uh, pfff££, I know we are recording but she she could actually receive an Oscar (.) because she can switch her emotions (.) immediately'. In this utterance, the clinician steps outside the frame of the discussion so far by making a meta-communicative statement. This appears to mark the importance he attaches to his statement, precisely because it would not normally be made as it is probably unprofessional and certainly controversial. This is a long speaking turn, compared to previous utterances and thereby illustrates that the clinician wants to make an important point for the development of his argument. This turn is then again mitigated by the same psychologist as before and reframes it by saying 'so when in a high level of stress and anxiety she might' (line 54). This attempt to soften the formulations about the mother is interrupted by the other clinician who says 'yes, yes, I am being very conscious of' (line 56). The interruption, the repetition of yes, as if that point from line 50 was somehow clear, is a form of dismissal of the softer description of the mother. Additionally, 'I am being very conscious of bringing that forward' as not to lose the important point he is making but also to forewarn the team who are about to take on the care of this service user.

Extract 2 firstly shows attempts to collaborate through initial questions to set the direction of the discussion. Secondly, it demonstrates extensions of turns are designed to support current state of discussions (Bolden, Mandelbaum, & Wilkinson, 2012). The lengthy and emotional outburst in the form of a rare meta-communicative statement by one clinician strengthens his contrasting position to the psychologists, who are attempting to mitigate formulations about the mother as being difficult.

Summary

The aim of this research was to identify psychological formulation discussions initiated by clinical psychologists in MDT learning disabilities meetings. There were three main outcomes of this project:

1. Psychological formulations were often not explicitly marked in the meeting discussions.
2. Where candidate exemplars were identifiable, they were marked by tentative pre-expansions (e.g. Extract 1: I guess I'm just struck that

...) which then combined general psychological theories with previous reports by colleagues and which in turn shaped healthcare professionals' understanding of the service users.

3. The analysis identified that delicate and sometimes emotional views of service users were expressed by healthcare professionals and psychological formulations came into the discussion to reframe these views in a more compassionate way.

The analysis of the MDT meetings highlighted a challenge in identifying psychological formulation in MDT discussions. The occasions when clinical psychologists 'chipped into' the discussion, then their contribution often did not follow the canonical format often attributed to formulations. When contributions which could be identified as psychological formulations did take place, the analysis suggested that they have an important role in shaping MDT members' understanding of service users' cases. The first exemplar of a psychological formulation in team discussions suggested that these are tentatively designed. The psychologist introduced the psychological concept as their own position by 'being struck by' or 'interested in' which links their eventual formulation to the case and grounds the formulation in the details of the case. Their formulation was constructed using general psychological concepts, such as 'children who have witnessed domestic violence experience emotional trauma' and were then linked with the information previously provided by other clinicians. The design of these formulations also supported the notion that psychologists are careful not to use jargon (Christofides et al., 2012) or impose their views.

The feature of designing the formulation by selecting, deleting and transforming the information provided by previous speakers has previously been illustrated in CA research on conversational formulations (Antaki et al., 2005; Bercelli et al., 2008). The formulation discussion serves to shape team members' understandings of service users' difficulties. This shift in understanding is also marked through change of state tokens (e.g. Extract 1, line 15: Yeah, oh yeah). This supports previous research that team formulation changes staff understanding of service users' mental health problems (Berry et al., 2009, Unadkat et al., 2015).

The analysis also suggested that psychological formulations were developed in order to present different and more compassionate perspectives on difficult service users (e.g. Extract 2: several team members had described a mother as difficult to work with). On this occasion, the psychologist initiates a turn which has an interrogative format and is valenced towards agreement. This turn also can be heard to make a bid for an extended turn and projects the line of argument that the extended turn will take. The bid for an extended turn also brought a collaborative element to the discussion. Some of the hypotheses that followed provided justifications for particular interventions, e.g. 'help the mother' to 'avoid her sabotaging' and perhaps to pre-empt disengagement. These hypotheses were extended at several points, perhaps working towards gaining the acceptance from others (Bolden & Angell, 2017). Other, much briefer formulations, reframed previous accounts to mitigate previous, less sympathetic hypotheses about the mother. Informal team formulation discussions can accommodate emotionally laden interactions.

Implications for Clinical Practice and Interprofessional Working

Given the difficulties in identifying psychological formulations in the data, it is likely that other mental health professionals would also struggle. Therefore, a recommendation for clinical practice would be to present more transparent formulation ideas (e.g. Hollingworth & Johnstone, 2014), e.g. by naming the psychological hypothesis and the reasons for including them in the discussion.

The priority seems to be given to the formulation by clinical psychologists which raises a question how other professionals experience the inclusion of their voices in these.

Tips for future research
• The use of discursive research (like CA) of dedicated formulation meetings may provide more information on the interactional formulation processes in MDT settings.
• Access to formulation meetings posed a significant challenge for this project, so source your participating teams in wide geographical areas.
• Larger samples may give more information on the structure and therefore defining features of team formulations.
• Team formulation meetings might offer more opportunity to record and analyse team processes as mentioned above as a feature of the psychologists' role and subsequently provide research evidence for these clinical practices.
• Keep re-evaluating the codes (e.g. is this code representative of a team formulation with both psychologists and researchers) as the characterisation of these is complicated and cross-checking improves the quality of the analysis.

References

Antaki, C., Barnes, R., & Leudar, I. (2005). Self-disclosure as a situated interactional practice. *British Journal of Social Psychology, 44*(2), 181–199. https://doi.org/10.1348/014466604x1573.

Bercelli, F., Rossano, F., & Viaro, M. (2008). Clients' responses to therapists' reinterpretations. In Perakyla, A. Antaki, C., Vehvilainen, S., & Leudar I. (Eds.), *Conversation analysis and psychotherapy.* Cambridge: Cambridge University Press.

Berry, K., Barrowclough, C., & Wearden, A. (2009). A pilot study investigating the use of psychological formulations to modify staff perceptions of service users with psychosis. *Behavioural and Cognitive Psychotherapy, 37,* 39–48.

Berry, K., Haddock, G., Kellett, S., Roberts, C., Drake, R., & Barrowclough, C. (2016). Feasibility of a ward-based psychological intervention to improve staff and patient relationships in psychiatric rehabilitation setting. *British Journal of Clinical Psychology, 55,* 236–252.

Bolden, G. B., & Angell, B. (2017). The organization of the treatment recommendation phase in routine psychiatric visits. *Research on Language and Social Interaction, 50*(2), 151–170. https://doi.org/10.1080/08351813.2017.1301299.

Bolden, G. B., Mandelbaum, J. S., & Wilkinson, S. (2012). Pursuing a response by repairing an indexical reference. *Research on Language and Social Interaction, 45*(2), 137–155.

Christofides, S., Johnstone, L., & Musa, M. (2012). 'Chippin in': Clinical psychologists' descriptions of their use of formulation in multidisciplinary team working. *Psychology and Psychotherapy; Theory, Research and Practice, 85,* 424–435.

Division of Clinical Psychology. (2010). *The core purpose and the philosophy of the profession.* Leicester: The British Psychological Society.

Fitzgerald P. (2013). *Therapy talk: Conversation analysis in practice.* Basingstoke: Palgrave Macmillan. https://doi.org/10.1057/9781137329530.

Heritage, J. (1984). A change-of-state token and aspects of its sequential placement. In J. M. Atkinson & J. Heritage (Eds.), *Structures of social action: Studies in conversation analysis* (pp. 299–344). Cambridge: Cambridge University Press.

Heritage, J., & Clayman, S. (2010). *Talk in action: Interactions, identities, and institutions.* Oxford: Wiley.

Heritage, J., & Watson, R. (1979). Formulations as conversational objects. In G. Psathas (Ed.), *Everyday language: Studies in ethnomethodology* (pp. 123–162). New York: Irvington.

Hollingworth, P., & Johnstone, L. (2014). Team formulation: What are the staff views? *Clinical Psychology Forum, 257*(5), 28–34.

Hood, N., Johnstone, L., & Christofides, S. (2013). The hidden solution? Staff experiences, views and understanding of the use of psychological formulation in multi-disciplinary teams. *The Journal of Critical Psychology, Counselling and Psychotherapy, 13*(2).

Ingham, B., & Clarke, L. (2009). The introduction of clinical psychology services to an inpatient autistic spectrum disorders and intellectual disabilities service: Impact and reflections. *Clinical Psychology Forum, 204,* 30–34.

Johnstone, L. (2014). Using formulations in teams. In L. Johnstone & R. Dallos (Eds.), *Formulation in psychology and psychotherapy, making sense of people's problems.* London: Routledge.

Johnstone, L., & Dallos, R. (2014). *Formulation in psychology and psychotherapy, making sense of people's problems* (2nd ed.). Routledge: London.

Pillet-Shore, D. (2010). Making way and making sense: Including newcomers in interaction. *Social Psychology Quarterly, 73*(2), 152–175.

QSR International's NVivo 11 Software, QSR International Pty Ltd. Version 11.

Summers, A. (2006). Psychological formulations in psychiatric care: Staff views on their impact. *Psychiatric Bulletin, 30,* 341–343.

Tileaga, C, & Stokoe, E. (2015). *Discursive psychology: Classic and contemporary issues.* Abingdon: Routledge.

Unadkat, S., Irving Quinn, G., Jones, F. W., & Casares, P. (2015). Staff experiences of formulating within a team setting. *Clinical Psychology Forum, 275,* 85–88. ISSN 1757-2142 (Extended Online Edition).

8

Does This Child Have Autism? Exploring Team Discussions When Diagnosing Autistic Spectrum Disorder

Nicole Parish

Introduction

Autistic spectrum disorder (ASD) is challenging to diagnose, because other difficulties can 'mimic' its symptoms (Basu & Parry, 2013). There is currently a debate as to whether ASD is being over-diagnosed, since there is a high chance of obtaining a false-positive result (Basu & Parry, 2013). To address this complexity, changes have been made to the diagnostic criteria of ASD (Basu & Parry, 2013). It is recommended that ASD is assessed for in children by a multidisciplinary team (MDT) rather than one clinician (Le Couteur, 2003; NICE, 2011), as it is considered to be a more reliable diagnostic decision-making process than that of independent clinicians (Westman Andersson, Miniscalco, & Gillberg, 2013). With this recommendation, the use of MDT

N. Parish (✉)
Child Health Psychology, Cardiff and Vale University
Health Board, Cardiff, UK
e-mail: Nicole.Parish@wales.nhs.uk

© The Author(s) 2018
C. Smart and T. Auburn (eds.), *Interprofessional Care and Mental Health*,
The Language of Mental Health, https://doi.org/10.1007/978-3-319-98228-1_8

assessments has increased in the UK; only 48% of child development teams used an MDT approach to assess for ASD in 2001, rising to 93% in 2007 (Palmer, Ketteridge, Parr, Baird, & Le Couteur, 2011).

To further enhance the reliability of diagnosing ASD, psycho-metric assessments can be helpful, yet it is recommended that they should be used with caution since they are vulnerable to interpre-tative bias (Falkmer, Anderson, Falkmer, & Horlin, 2013). A sys-tematic review concluded that a combination of tools could yield a diagnostic accuracy of 80.8% (Falkmer et al., 2013). This high accu-racy rate is seen as 'gold standard', yet it implies that the tools are not accurate for one in five cases. It is suggested that whilst psychometric assessments can be useful, they must always be used alongside clinical judgement.

As part of the diagnostic process, clinicians are also encouraged to explore whether ASD is the most appropriate way of understanding a child's difficulties. NICE (2011) lists 17 difficulties that can commonly be mistaken for ASD that should be considered, including specific lan-guage difficulties, hearing impairments, anxiety and attachment difficul-ties. Whilst this list can help clinicians to identify possible alternatives, it does not inform clinicians of how to differentiate between the dif-ferent possibilities. Basu and Parry (2013) recommend developing a bio-psycho-social formulation to help understand a child's difficulties: exploring how issues such as social anxiety, developmental trauma and attachment difficulties may have influenced a child's development. Moran (2010) discussed why a child with developmental trauma and/or attachment difficulties may present with ASD type symptoms and noted subtle differences that clinicians can look out for. For example, Moran writes:

> *Children on the autism spectrum and those with attachment problems both present difficulty with flexible thinking and behaviour… The need for pre-dictability in attachment disorder suggests that the child is trying to have their emotional needs for security and identity met. In autism, the emphasis seems to be on trying to make the world fit with the child's preferences. (Moran, 2010, p. 50)*

Think point
• When teams assess for autism, they should also consider other explanations for a child's presentation, within the context of their early experiences.

It seems that one way of enabling an MDT assessment is for different clinicians to conduct independent assessments with a child and family, and then to meet as a team to discuss the results within a professionals-only post-assessment meeting. These meetings provide a forum in which teams can collate the information gathered and explore whether or not to give a child an ASD diagnosis. To investigate these ASD post-assessment meetings, Bartolo, Dockrell, and Lunt (2001) audio-recorded the discussions of 4 children being assessed for ASD and analysed the meetings using content analysis. It was found that an MDT meeting provided a space for 'thinking-out-loud' hypothesis testing for the clinicians. A six-stage nonlinear model of decision-making was proposed, which included describing the problem, explaining the problem and making a plan of action.

Yet, as Bartolo et al. (2001) themselves acknowledged, the interpersonal processes of these meetings could not be explored with content analysis. Therefore, the study could not establish how interactions between the team members may have impacted on the discussions—for example how clinicians negotiated different possibilities and/or perceptions (or not). It could be argued that the findings are therefore an over simplistic representation of what occurs within post-assessment meetings, which does not go far enough in investigating the complex process of diagnosis as an *interactional* achievement. Conducting a similar study using conversation analysis (CA), on the other hand, would capture interactional processes and the subtle variations in talk that can alter its implied meaning (Sidnell, 2010). The sentence 'I don't think he has ASD', for example, may be said in different ways. An emphasis on 'I' may suggest that the person is giving his/her own account, perhaps in contrast to someone else's. An emphasis on 'think' may suggest uncertainty of their opinion. Whereas an emphasis on 'ASD' might imply that the person thinks the child has a difficulty, but it may not be

ASD. Yet, ASD post-assessment team meetings do not appear to have been explored in this way before.

Research conducted in broader healthcare, non-ASD, settings has begun to reveal the interactional complexities of MDT meetings. For example, Kidger, Murdoch, Donovan, and Blazeby (2009) found that clinicians from different disciplines focused on different information within a gynaecological oncology setting; nurses were more likely to focus on patient-related factors than the consultant oncologists, who focused more on disease-related information. Additionally, research has shown that different team members may have different levels of influence in meetings. Seniority may increase one's influence (Kidger et al., 2009)—as might, having met the person being discussed (Dew, Stubbe, Signal, Stairmand, Dennett, Koea, 2014). Furthermore, factors other than the team members themselves can impact on the interpersonal process of MDT meetings. These include the organisational structure, the complexity of the patient's needs and the preparation time available to clinicians (Croker, Loftus, & Higgs, 2008; Kidger et al., 2009; Sarkar, Arora, Lamb, Green, Sevdalis, & Dazi, 2014). Nonetheless, team meetings can provide a safe space to question practices and negotiate boundaries (Arber, 2007).

Implications for interprofessional working

- Clinicians from different disciplines focus on different information during team meetings.
- Having met the person being discussed, or having time to prepare for the meeting, also influences the contributions made by clinicians.

Given the complexities of MDT meetings on a general level, and the emphasis on MDT-based assessments in ASD, it seems pertinent to explore the discussions of teams diagnosing ASD. The current study aimed to investigate how teams explore whether or not to give a child an ASD diagnosis during post-assessment meetings.

Project Overview

Design

Naturalistic data was obtained by recording meetings in which MDTs discussed children who had recently been assessed for ASD. Only clinicians were present at these meetings, the child and/or family were not. The purpose of these meetings was to decide whether or not to give each child discussed a diagnosis of ASD, based on information gathered from multiple assessments independently conducted by clinicians in the MDT.

Recruitment

Four tertiary specialist ASD[1] services were invited to take part. Services were included that:

- assessed children for ASD;
- used a multidisciplinary approach;
- routinely discussed the assessment outcomes in an MDT meeting;
- worked within, or on behalf of, the National Health Service (NHS); and
- were based within a specific locality.

Tips for doing research

- Following advice from service users and the National Research Ethics Service, the families of the children being discussed in the meetings were not informed about the research. To ensure anonymity, identifiable information was replaced with white noise on the recordings and details of the teams and/or families were not transcribed.
---

[1]The services referred to themselves as ASC services, since they preferred the term autistic spectrum condition. The term ASD has been used, however, for consistency within the literature.

Prior to selection, it was decided that teams would be excluded if they were considered to be in a state of undue uncertainty, change or stress, in order to minimise any potential negative impacts of the research. No services approached were excluded based on this criterion, however.

The manager of each service was contacted, and information was sent via email to the teams. From this, two services expressed an interest in participating. The author visited these services to discuss the study with all members of the teams. Participants were given a week to consider the project, after which they all consented to take part. Team A consented to audio recording of the meetings and Team B consented to both audio and video recording.

Data Collection

The meetings were audio and/or video recorded depending on the teams' preference. This method enabled the collection of 'naturally occurring' talk (Potter & Hepburn, 2005). Recording equipment was given to a designated member of the team prior to the meeting, who was responsible for setting up the equipment and recording the data.

Three half-day meetings were recorded from the two multidisciplinary teams (two meetings from Team A and one from Team B). This captured the discussions of 16 children across 8 hours 24 minutes of data (6 children and 4 hours 46 minutes hours from Team A; 10 children and 3 hours and 39 minutes from Team B).

Participants

The participants were staff members of the two MDTs. The clinicians introduced themselves at the start of the meetings being recorded, saying their name and job title. The professional groups included clinical psychology, educational psychology, speech and language therapy, nursing and paediatric medicine. At the meetings, there were also team members with role titles that did not define a professional body, such as

ASD practitioners, managerial staff and admin staff. The role of the clinicians, however, has not been factored into the analysis.

The two teams held the meetings in slightly different ways. Team A held weekly meetings over half a day. Clinicians would come in and out of the meeting, to be present for the discussions of the children on their caseload. Team A's meetings varied from 3 to 5 clinicians in size. Team B held monthly meetings over half a day. The team reported that the meetings were less frequent than they would wish because many of the clinicians worked on a part-time basis for the ASD service. Within these meetings, the clinicians would stay for the entirety of the meeting and were present for the discussions of all the children. The size of Team B meetings varied between 9 and 11 clinicians.

Data Analysis

Conversation analysis was applied to the data (Sidnell, 2010). First, the meetings were transcribed orthographically. During this, ideas for potential areas of analysis were generated. The discussion of psychometric assessments was identified as a particularly rich area for further exploration, as the clinicians compared the objective scores with their subjective opinions. The conversations regarding psychometric assessments were therefore chosen as a focus of analysis.

Sections of the data discussing psychometric assessments were gathered by listening to the recordings and searching the transcripts. Twenty-four extracts were collated and transcribed using the Jeffersonian conventions (Jefferson, 2004). These extracts were repeatedly listened to and detailed notes were made about the talk, including intonations, utterances and silences. A summary of around 400–500 words was written for each extract. From these, the author explored what occurred within the sequences, such as how topics were started and how the conversation progressed. Interesting features were investigated further, focusing on what happened in the conversation after such a feature occurred.

Data Credibility

Extracts from the data were taken to a CA data analysis group. This enhanced the validity of the analysis by gaining multiple perspectives. Additionally, the author engaged in bracketing interviews before data collection and during the data analysis stage (Rolls & Relf, 2006). This is a process in which one acknowledges, or 'brackets off', subjective assumptions in an attempt to reduce the impact of these in the analysis. For this, the author was interviewed by a colleague about the project, specifically questioning about assumptions, feelings or personal connections to the topic. These interviews were recorded and transcribed, so they could be referred back to at set times points, such as after the initial data analysis.

Analysis

This study examined how MDTs explore whether to give a child an ASD diagnosis during post-assessment meetings. The analysis revealed conversational practices that encouraged the team to elaborate on information. This included building on, clarifying or querying information (collectively referred to here as elaboration). This 'opened up' the discussion, creating space to explore possible accounts for a child's presentation, including ASD and non-ASD alternatives—here termed 'candidate suggestions'.[2]

Whilst there may be many ways to open up a discussion, this analysis focused on three specific practices observed within the data. These were: presenting information in an uncertain manner; interjecting a discussion to present relevant information; and responding to information

---

[2]Adapted from term *'candidate explanation'*, Pomerantz et al. (2007) used to describe how patients give possible explanations for an illness. 'Candidate suggestions' is here used because the suggestions did not appear to be offered as a definitive explanation, but as a possible consideration.

in a way that displays its noteworthiness. These practices appeared to encourage clinicians to elaborate on information, even in time-limited meetings. Overlaps in the practices were observed; for example, responding with noteworthiness could be identified in combination with the other two.

In addition to these practices, interesting differences were found in the way the clinicians discussed the candidate suggestions. It seemed that some candidate suggestions were more sensitive for the clinicians to talk about than others.

Presenting Information with Uncertainty

Within this practice, a team member would present information in a way that indicated confusion or uncertainty. This was done through increased hesitation, elongated words and pauses in the talk. The display of uncertainty appeared to give space for elaboration, in which clinicians could explore different candidate suggestions.

Extract 1. From Team B[3]

```
1   Anne        sh:e (.) scored on 3DI based on
2        →      <mother's report> a:::nd e:r
3        →      (0.8) s:he did ↑not score on
4        →      ↓ADOS
5   Sam  →      Hmm
```

---

[3]Pseudonyms have been used throughout, including those within the talk.

```
6    Claire   →   ↑Oh

7    Anne         and Lucy was (.) >er< at the

8                 end of the clinic sh- she was

9                 like (.) *she's=a

10               *totally=different [*girl]=

11   Claire                        [Ha ha]

12   Anne        =from what I saw <at> <home>

13   Claire      Oh re↑ally

14   Debra       ↑Oh

15   Anne        so it was good that you saw her

16               a(h)t

17               ho(h)me and that you did the

18        →      ADOS so um (.) so we were not

19        →      sure whether it:s (.) anxiety or

20        →      is it autism

21   Claire  →   Has she had a scho:ol (.) o:bs

22               of any sort

23   Anne        no

24   Claire      Okay

25   Anne        that=that was the thi:ng that

26               was missing

27   Sam         I think there's something (.)

28               there's been some question in

29               the past about (.)

30        →      °<fabricated>° °<illness>°=
```

```
31   Anne:        =in the past when she was

32                younger there were hmm

33   Debra        O:h↓ don't (think of) that then

35   Claire       Parental fabricated or her

35                fabricated parental? Parental
```

Here, Anne informs the team about how a child scored on two psychometric assessments: 3DI (Developmental, Dimensional and Diagnostic Interview) and ADOS (Autism Diagnostic Observation Schedule). Anne slows down as she says 'mother's report', as if to emphasise it (line 2). There is then a pause of 0.8 seconds before she says 'she did not score on ADOS' (lines 3 and 4). This hesitation, along with an upward intonation and emphasis on 'not', appears to signal trouble. The team members responded to this in a way that indicates it is newsworthy ('Hmm' and 'Oh', lines 5 and 6). Anne again indicates uncertainty by stating 'we are not sure' (lines 18 and 19) followed by two candidate suggestions of 'anxiety' or 'autism' (lines 19 and 20).

This display of uncertainty appears to create a space for elaboration. In this, Claire asks about a 'school obs' (observations) (line 21), presumably in an attempt to gather more information. Sam then appears to imply an additional candidate suggestion by saying there has previously been fabricated illness (line 30). The conversation that follows suggests that, by this, Claire is questioning the validity of the mother's report.

Interjecting

A discussion could also be opened up by a clinician 'interjecting', here defined as interrupting a discussion with relevant information. A clinician's interjection was responded to in a way that demonstrated the information had been relevant, which created a space for further elaboration. Within this, candidate suggestions could be explored.

Extract 2. From Team B

1	Anne	→	the ↑difficulty i:s that ↑h:e h:as
2		→	sc:ored o::n (.) both the ↓to::ols
3	Alex		Yes
4	Claire		Mmmm
5	Anne		>yes I know< >its< it's um mer
6			repo:rt (.) >parental re↓po:rt< (.)
7			↑scho:ol are obs are are not e:x
8			very saying no not at ↓al::l=
9	Alex	→	=But but<Jenny saw him=
10	Anne	→	[an:d]
11	Alex	→	=[in ↑school] and
12		→	said no=
13	Claire		=saying no no as well
14	Anne		you saw him in [↑scho:ol]
15	Jenny		[I I]
16	Anne		or just (.) alright (.) I thought
17	Jenny		I saw him in school and I completed
18			a >speech and language< assessment
19			with him as we:ll
20	Anne		alright so you

21	Jenny		yeah
22	Anne		didn't s::ee an::y
23	Jenny		I didn't n:o and I'm<I haven't looked
24			through the ADOS but I'm just
25			<u>wondering</u> if he's scored on <u>that</u> (.)
26			because of this lack of kind of
27			social receprocity
28	Alex		that's what I was thinking
29	Jenny		which is quite <u>common</u> with children
30			that are presenting how ↑he ↑was
31		→	he has quite a low self esteem
32			and he's not (.) can't be bothered
33			really hh
34	Alex	→	very very feels like anxiety (.)
35			>social anxiety<
36	Claire		yeah
37	Kat		°Mmm°

This extract follows a discussion about a boy whose psychometric assessments suggest ASD, but his speech and language profile did not. Anne appears to imply that there is not enough evidence to reject ASD (lines 1–8). She presents this as a 'difficulty' (line 1), explaining that 'he has scored on both the tools' (suggesting ASD) (lines 1 and 2) and that the school observation had not indicated 'no' ASD (lines 6–8). Alex then interjects (lines 9 and 11). This appears to be a pre-emptory claim for the floor as it comes at a TCU (see Chapter 2) where Anne has not given an indication of stopping her turn or selecting another speaker (Schegloff, 2007); where speakers make a pre-emptory claim for the floor or interrupt an ongoing TCU, this often displays a project of altering the trajectory of the talk in progress. This shifted trajectory is marked by the contrastive connective (line 9: 'but'). It is done to inform Anne that 'Jenny saw him in school and said no [ASD]' (lines 9–12). This is new and relevant information, as Anne responds with 'you saw him in school', with a high intonation on school as a repeat newsmarker (line 14). The direction of the conversation seems to change following this interjection, in a way that opens up the discussion for elaboration. Following this, three candidate suggestions are discussed: lack of reciprocity (lines 26–27), low self-esteem (line 31) and social anxiety (line 35).

Responding with Noteworthiness

In this particularly prevalent practice, team members responded to information in a way that suggested it was relevant, here termed responding with noteworthiness. This was done, for example, by showing surprise through talking with a high intonation. Yet, noteworthy information did not always appear surprising, as some information seemed to be of note but not unexpected. This was demonstrated, for example, by repeating a word after someone else had said it. When team members responded to information with noteworthiness, it appeared to create an opening for elaboration. Within this, candidate suggestions could be explored.

Extract 3. From Team A

```
1    Michelle   So that wa:s (.) the ADOS↓.

2    Hannah  →  =and he sco:red quite [highly]

3    Michelle                         [He:   ]

4               h:as ↑yeah

5    Phillip →  Mmm, seventeen

6    Hannah  →  Seventeen over all [wasn't it]

7    Michelle→                     [Seventeen]

8               yeah   overall

9    David   →  Over↑all sevente↑en was ↑it

10   Hannah     Well yeah

11   Michelle   I mean pa:rt of that (.) high

12              sco:re I think could be

13           →  explained by his reticence↓ and

14           →  his shyness↓

15   Hannah     Ye:ah

16   Michelle   And

17   Karen   →  =And also his speech and

18           →  language communication

19           →  [difficul↑ties]

20   Michelle   [yes]          Ye:s ye:s he was

21              looking for words (.) he was (.)

22              and he needed ti:me to pr:ocess
```

Michelle had previously summarised a child's performance on an assessment (ADOS). This is followed by Hannah adding that the child had 'scored quite highly' (line 2) and the assessment score of 'seventeen' is given by Phillip (line 5). The number 'seventeen' is then repeated three more times (lines 6, 7, and 9), displaying surprise. In addition, when David repeats 'seventeen' he does so with an upward intonation and 'was it' at the end, both signifying surprise (line 9). This surprise suggests that the information was relevant and noteworthy. The response of noteworthiness gives space for elaboration. Within this, two candidate suggestions are given by Michelle of 'reticence' and 'shyness' (lines 13 and 14) and a third by Karen of 'speech and language communication difficulties' (lines 17–19).

Think point

- Information could be presented, or responded to, in a way that encouraged the team to elaborate on it. This created a space to explore different explanations for a child's presentation, including alternatives to ASD.

How Candidate Suggestions Were Discussed

When analysing the above three practices, differences were noticed in the way candidate suggestions were discussed. Some appeared to be said with ease, shown by the speaker voicing the candidate suggestion without any hesitation. In Extract 3, for example, Karen suggests that the high score on a child's assessment may be associated with 'his speech and language communication difficulties' (lines 17–19). This follows on from the previous line without any apparent hesitation. In contrast, some candidate suggestions appeared to be talked about in a more tentative way, as though they were more sensitive or 'delicate' issues (Silverman & Peräkylä, 1990). This was shown by difficulties in the talk before the candidate suggestion was voiced (Silverman & Peräkylä, 1990). In Extract 1, for example, Sam builds up to the words 'fabricated illness' by saying 'I think there's something, there's been some question in the past about' (lines 27–30). There are also pauses in the talk and the term 'fabricated illness' is said quieter than the rest of the sentence. This makes it seem as though the candidate suggestion of fabricated illness is a sensitive issue—more so, perhaps, than 'speech and language communication difficulties'.

Think point

- Some explanations of a child's behaviour seemed to be more sensitive to discuss than others.

Discussion

This study aimed to explore meetings in which MDTs consider whether or not to give a child an ASD diagnosis after an assessment. Prior to this study, there had been a paucity of research regarding post-assessment meetings. Specific conversational practices were identified that encouraged clinicians to elaborate on information that had been presented. This provided an opportunity to discuss different accounts for a child's presentation (candidate suggestions), including ASD and non-ASD alternatives. Three practices were identified: presenting information in an uncertain manner; interjecting a discussion to present relevant information; and responding to information in a way that suggests it was noteworthy. Additionally, it appeared that some possible accounts for a child's presentation were more sensitive to discuss than others.

Recommendations for Interprofessional Working

Demystifying the process of an ASD assessment is in itself beneficial, as is highlighting the complex and subjective nature of diagnosing ASD. It appeared that holding an MDT meeting as a routine part of an ASD assessment gave space for different accounts of a child's presentation to be explored (also see Chapter 12 on 'concern constructions'). As discussed in the Introduction, there is a risk of over-diagnosing ASD (Basu & Parry, 2013). Since MDT meetings seem to help clinicians elaborate on information and explore alternative explanations, their use may reduce the likelihood of a false-positive diagnosis. This could have multiple benefits. Firstly, direct benefits for the children being assessed for ASD and their families, as understanding what's going on is the first step in offering the right support (Moran, 2010). More widely, it could lessen the societal impacts of over-diagnosing ASD, such as an increased demand for limited resources and pressures on the welfare system (Basu & Parry, 2013).

The findings revealed conversational practices that encourage clinicians to elaborate on information within MDT meetings. Such practices could be used for training or reflective practice in MDT working. The benefits of opening up discussions to enable all voices from the MDT to be heard could be highlighted to clinicians chairing meetings. On the other hand, less assertive clinicians, who may find it difficult to present their opinions, could be shown how even slight utterances, such as a surprised 'oh', can change the direction of a conversation.

Additionally, highlighting the benefits of team meetings can be helpful in evidencing their necessity. This is particularly needed in times of austerity, when services are under pressure to provide a high standard of care in less time and with fewer resources. This study could demonstrate that face-to-face meetings are an integral part of a clinician's role that may enhance MDT working.

An MDT assessment of ASD is considered as more reliable than that of a single clinician (Westman Andersson et al., 2013). The current findings may start to account for why this might be. For these teams, it appeared that discussing the results as an MDT encouraged information to be elaborated on. This created space for clinicians to consider multiple options of a child's presentation, including biological, psychological and social factors. Suggestions of anxiety, shyness and communication difficulties were considered, for example. Exploring such alternatives to ASD may reduce the likelihood of a false-positive diagnosis (Basu & Parry, 2013).

Moreover, there may be bespoke qualities that the face-to-face contact within a meeting provides, which other forms of MDT communication, such as submitting written reports, could not. Perhaps such a rich elaboration and consideration would not have occurred if a single clinician were to form the diagnostic decision based on written information from the MDT, without opportunity for discussion. Such a method would still meet the guidelines of an MDT assessment, but would create a very different pathway than that of an MDT post-assessment meeting. The analysis revealed conversational practices that prompted the clinicians to elaborate on a point and/or to give candidate suggestions for it. This elaborating on information may not have occurred if the clinician did not get instantaneous feedback from the team members in the meeting.

An MDT meeting may help to lessen the confirmation biases of any one clinician, since it creates space to consider multiple possible accounts for a child's presentation. We are all prone to focusing on information that confirms our beliefs and discounting information that does not. This may limit a clinician's ability to look for alternative accounts when assessing for ASD. It has been shown that clinicians looking for confirmatory evidence gave the 'wrong diagnoses' 70% of the time when assessing for general psychiatric conditions (Mendel, Traut-Mattausch, Jonas, Leucht, Kane, 2011). Additionally, McHoul and Rapley (2005) explored the diagnostic process of a paediatrician assessing a boy for attention-deficit/hyperactivity disorder (ADHD). The paediatrician focused on information that supported ADHD and discarded incongruent information. This resulted in a diagnosis of ADHD being given, despite there been conflicting evidence. Cognitive biases will filter what a clinician attends to during an assessment, which may lead them to focus more on information that confirms an ASD diagnosis. Having conversational cues within an MDT meeting that encourages elaboration may make clinicians more attentive to all relevant information. For example, if information had not been considered by the speaker, but was responded to with surprise from the team, it may make the clinician reconsider its relevance.

Another interesting finding was that some possible accounts for a child's presentation seemed more sensitive to voice than others. Such issues can be spoken about in an MDT meeting in a tentative way. The speaker is able to gauge from the team's response how the information is being received, and continue to discuss the point if it is deemed safe enough to do so. This would not be the case if information were submitted in a report, as something cannot be unwritten once it has been documented. Clinicians may therefore feel able to question uncertainties in a sensitive way within a meeting, such as suspicions of abuse or neglect, which they may not otherwise raise. It is essential that clinicians feel able to consider such possibilities, not only for the diagnostic outcome but also for the welfare of the child. MDT meetings seem to provide clinicians with freedom to tentatively explore ideas without them being misconstrued as fact.

The team meetings provided space for psychometric assessments to be elaborated upon, but interestingly this was done in different ways. Clinicians in Team A would routinely read through each assessment, giving a sense of what the child was like and how they performed. For this team, it appeared that this qualitative description was as important as the score. The clinicians in Team B, however, were more likely to present only the score or outcome of an assessment. Though assessments were presented in this way, conversational practices frequently led to further elaboration. Thus, the elaboration of the psychometric assessments was common, even if only the score had initially been presented. It appeared that clinicians were not only focusing on either the test scores or their clinical perceptions, but that the consideration of one led naturally onto the other.

Further Research

Whilst CA explored what and how things were said, it did not offer interpretations of the wider societal and contextual meanings. It was found that some candidate suggestions were more difficult to discuss than others; however, this study was limited in its ability to explore why this might be. There may be societal influences, for example, that have an impact on how 'delicate' a candidate suggestion is to discuss. Over recent years, the stigma of autism appears to have lessened and it is widely considered to have a biological origin, and hence withholds parental 'blame' or responsibility. ASD may therefore seem more socially acceptable than other possible accounts of a child's difficulties, such as those relating to attachment difficulties or abuse. It would be interesting to explore this, by using an additional form of analysis, such as critical discourse analysis.

From this study, it seemed that elaboration would lead to a more considered diagnostic decision, although it could not establish whether conversational practices had an impact on the outcome. There were examples where the conversational practices seemed to change the trajectory of the conversations, which could potentially alter the diagnostic decision. Future research could empirically consider whether opening up discussions does have an impact on the final diagnostic outcomes.

Summary

It appears that MDT meetings provide a space for clinicians to explore different accounts for a child's presentation after an ASD assessment. There were specific conversational practices that encouraged clinicians to elaborate on information. It is questioned whether such rich discussions would have been had if the MDT meetings had not been a routine part of the ASD assessments. The finding of this study, in addition to future research, could help to make recommendations on MDT practices when assessing children for ASD, potentially reducing the risk of over-diagnosing ASD.

Acknowledgements   Firstly, I would like to thank the two teams that took part in this study. I appreciate how exposing it must have been to have someone record their work and they demonstrated great practices in collaborative team working. Secondly, I would like to thank my supervisors: Cordet Smart for her encouragement and enthusiasm throughout, and Jacqui Stedmon for her calming and reflective influence. Finally, I would also like to say a big thank you to Dr Lindsay Aikman for all of your help and support.

References

Arber, A. (2007). "Pain talk" in hospice and palliative care team meetings: An ethnography. *International Journal of Nursing Studies, 44,* 916–926.

Bartolo, P. A., Dockrell, J., & Lunt, I. (2001). Naturalistic decision-making task processes in multiprofessional assessment of disability. *Journal of School Psychology, 39,* 499–519.

Basu, S., & Parry, P. (2013). The autism spectrum disorder 'epidemic': Need for biopsychosocial formulation. *Australian and New Zealand Journal of Psychiatry, 47,* 1116–1118.

Croker, A, Loftus, S., & Higgs, J. (2008). Multidisciplinary clinical decision making. In *Clinical reasoning in the health professions* (pp. 291–298). Amsterdam: Butterworth-Heinemann.

Dew, K., Stubbe, M., Signal, L., Stairmand, J., Dennett, E., Koea J., …, Ellison-Loschmann, L. (2014) Cancer care decision making in multidisciplinary meetings. *Qualitative Health Research, 25*(3), 397–407.

Falkmer, T., Anderson, K., Falkmer, M., & Horlin, C. (2013). Diagnostic procedures in autism spectrum disorders: A systematic literature review. *European Child and Adolescent Psychiatry, 22,* 329–340.

Jefferson, G. (2004). Glossary of transcript symbols with an introduction. *Pragmatics and Beyond New Series, 125,* 13–34.

Kidger, J., Murdoch, J., Donovan, J. L., & Blazeby, J. M. (2009). Clinical decision-making in a multidisciplinary gynaecological cancer team: A qualitative study. *An International Journal of Obstetrics & Gynaecology, 116,* 511–517.

Le Couteur, A. (2003). *National Autism Plan for Children (NAPC): Plan for the identification, assessment, diagnosis and access to early interventions for pre-school and primary school aged children with autism spectrum disorders (ASD).* London: National Autistic Society.

McHoul, A., & Rapley, M. (2005). A case of attention-deficit/hyperactivity disorder diagnosis: Sir Karl and Francis B. slug it out on the consulting room floor. *Discourse & Society, 16,* 419–449.

Mendel, R., Traut-Mattausch, E., Jonas, E., Leucht, S., Kane, J. M., Maino, K., …, Hamann J. (2011). Confirmation bias: Why psychiatrists stick to wrong preliminary diagnoses. *Psychological Medicine, 41,* 2651–2659.

Moran, H. (2010). Clinical observations of the differences between children on the autism spectrum and those with attachment problems: The Coventry Grid. *Good Autism Practice (GAP), 11,* 46–59.

National Institute for Health and Care Excellence (NICE). (2011). Autism diagnosis in children and young people: Recognition, referral and diagnosis of children and young people on the autism spectrum. In *NICE clinical guidance* (p. 128). Manchester: NICE.

Palmer, E., Ketteridge, C., Parr, J. R., Baird, G., & Le Couteur, A. (2011). Autism spectrum disorder diagnostic assessments: Improvements since publication of the National Autism Plan for Children. *Archives of Disease in Childhood, 96,* 473–475.

Potter, J., & Hepburn, A. (2005). Qualitative interviews in psychology: Problems and possibilities. *Qualitative Research in Psychology, 2,* 281–307.

Rolls, L., & Relf, M. (2006). Bracketing interviews: Addressing methodological challenges in qualitative interviewing in bereavement and palliative care. *Mortality, 11,* 286–305.

Sarkar, S., Arora, S., Lamb, B. W., Green, J. S., Sevdalis, N., & Darzi, A. (2014). Case review in urology multidisciplinary team meetings: What members think of its functioning. *Journal of Clinical Urology, 7,* 394–402.

Schegloff, E. A. (2007). *Sequence organization in interaction: Volume 1: A primer in conversation analysis.* Cambridge: Cambridge University Press.

Sidnell, J. (2010). *Conversation analysis: An introduction.* Chichester: Wiley-Blackwell.

Silverman, D., & Peräkylä, A. (1990). AIDS counselling: The interactional organisation of talk about 'delicate' issues. *Sociology of Health & Illness, 12,* 293–318.

Westman Andersson G., Miniscalco, C., & Gillberg, C. (2013). Autism in preschoolers: Does individual clinician's first visit diagnosis agree with final comprehensive diagnosis? *The Scientific World Journal, 2013,* 1–7.

9

Negotiating Resources During CMHT Team Meetings: Exploring Requests for Joint Working

Sifiso Mhlanga and Timothy Auburn

Introduction

This chapter examines how staff working in Community Mental Health Teams (CMHTs) enlist the support of each other through making requests for joint working. When an individual comes into contact with community mental health services, the level of support that they require is devised collaboratively between the service user and a health care professional usually a Community Mental Health Nurse (CMHN). This process enables clinicians to take into account the individual's needs and the level of risk that they present with, whilst also considering other factors, such as their history of engaging with services and whether they require care coordination (Department of Health, 2002). Meeting the holistic needs of an individual

S. Mhlanga (✉)
Leicestershire Partnership Trust, Leicester, UK
e-mail: sifiso.mhlanga@nhs.net

T. Auburn
School of Psychology, University of Plymouth, Plymouth, UK
e-mail: T.Auburn@plymouth.ac.uk

© The Author(s) 2018
C. Smart and T. Auburn (eds.), *Interprofessional Care and Mental Health*,
The Language of Mental Health, https://doi.org/10.1007/978-3-319-98228-1_9

often requires input from other professionals. It is therefore common and best practice for clinicians to work jointly with other professionals within a multidisciplinary team (MDT). This often involves seeking an expert opinion, conducting a joint assessment or referring the service user for a specific intervention with another clinician within the team.

Internal referrals are routinely discussed in MDT meetings. Discussions about the service user's needs during MDT meetings often presents a dilemma for clinicians, as they are acutely aware of the needs of the individuals that they are supporting, as well as the pressures that the service is facing due to gaps within service provision. In 2002, the Department of Health recommended that CMHTs manage caseloads of up to 300–350 individuals, whilst full-time CMHN's can expect to manage individual caseloads of up to 35 individuals (Department of Health, 2002). However, more recently, some CMHNs working in services across the UK are managing caseloads of up to 49 individuals, with varying levels of complexity and need (Butler, 2005; Independent Mental Health Taskforce to NHS England, 2016). Whilst joint working is at the core of interdisciplinary and interagency working, many services are under-resourced and simply do not have the capacity or staffing resources to meet all of the needs of the service users.

Allocation meetings enable individual clinicians to share accountability with other team members, through requesting the involvement of others in the service user's recovery, thus ensuring effective team working (West, 1994). In a discursive study of CMHT allocation meetings, Griffiths (2001) found that specialist services were more likely to be offered to service users when clinicians (e.g. psychiatrists) used explicit diagnostic labels. In contrast, other clinicians (e.g. CMHNs and social workers) used implicit descriptions, that is a clinical formulation of mental health needs, as they offered a "less threatening way to question psychiatrists' definitions" and to introduce "alternatives" to diagnoses (p. 697). This suggests that the fundamental differences in how clinicians present the service user's needs has different implications in the services that are offered. Other research has found that hospital-based mental health triage nurses may feel reluctant to make referrals to professionals within the community due to concerns that they may be perceived as "soft" and "less able to manage the risks associated with the triage role" (Sands, 2009, p. 306). This highlights the importance of interdisciplinary and interagency team working, to ensure that there are clear care pathways and that referrals are made in a timely manner.

These findings, coupled with the observations about increases in caseloads and resource limitations suggest that making requests for the involvement of other members of the CMHT has a number of associated difficulties. There is the risk that one is encroaching unreasonably on another's workload as well as the risk to personal reputation in so far as requesting support from others might lead to the inference that one is not able to fulfil one's professional role adequately. Against these risks is the assumed ethos of joint working and professional collaboration. How requests for support are managed may also have implications for the service user's care pathway.

Requesting as a Social Action

Requesting has been researched extensively within the conversation analytic tradition and has provided a means of exploring how people recruit others in order to gain their assistance and contribution to a task in progress (Kendrick & Drew, 2016; Zinken & Rossi, 2016). Requests usually follow a description of a difficulty that needs resolving which gives permission for others to offer their assistance (Kendrick & Drew, 2016). Requests typically emerge in adjacency pairs—that is, they emerge in close succession and in two parts, with the first part reflecting the initiation and the second part reflecting the response or outcome—approval or disapproval (Heritage & Clayman, 2010; Schegloff, 2006; see also Chapter 2). Responses to requests are dependent upon the participants' shared understanding of the wider context, for example the contingencies (the ability of the person to fulfil the request) within the health care setting, as well as the availability of resources (e.g. staffing levels and caseload capacities).

Recent work in CA has also identified how participants display, in the way that they design their requests what they understand as the relevant dimensions of the social context. Curl and Drew (2008) argue that interrogative and declarative requests are commonly used in institutional settings as they address differences in authority (entitlement) and contingencies. This suggests that conversation analysis may offer several ways in which issues related to resources and caseload capacities might be negotiated through the clinicians' talk during allocation meetings. One strategy that clinicians may use is through including pre-requests ("do you have capacity?") in their speech. Pre-requests provide the person initiating the request with key information that may guide them as to whether or not to proceed with the request (Fox, 2015). As such, conversation analysis may offer practical guidance for health care professionals on how to articulate and enlist the assistance of others within the current context of limited resources.

The aim of this chapter is to explore how clinicians initiated and designed requests for joint working during CMHT allocation meetings. This chapter will also examine how the requests were responded to by other members of the MDT, in particular, the chair of the meetings who is often the team manager, given the current context where there are pressures to gatekeep services due to limited resources. The chair is, by reference to their allocated role, in a pivotal position to grant or resist requests for support.

Project Overview

Background

I had just finished a year-long clinical psychology placement within a CMHT in the National Health Service (NHS) when I developed an interest in examining team allocation meetings. The local Mental health services where I had completed my placement had recently undergone a service redesign, and each CMHT had expanded in its catchment area and was now providing services to a wider population. There were several vacancies across the service for CMHNs, occupational therapists and other professionals. The service was under-resourced, and clinicians were managing higher caseloads in order to meet the needs of the service users within their growing catchment area. There had also been interest from the senior management team to explore the function of the weekly MDT allocation meetings, with a particular focus on the decision-making process that occurred during the allocation meetings.

The allocation meetings were held weekly and were attended by health professionals only. The allocation meetings offered a forum where clinicians could share their concerns about the well-being of an individual on their caseload |(see also Chapter 6), which opened up the space for clinicians to request input from other members of the MDT (e.g. joint assessment or specialist interventions). The meetings aimed to foster a team discussion about new referrals to be seen by the team which would shape the clinical decisions relating to the allocation of team resources, or indeed whether someone would benefit from a referral to another service due to a change in their risks and level of needs. Team managers typically had a background in nursing and had the responsibility for chairing the meetings.

Ethical approval was granted, and I arranged face-to-face meetings with managers of each catchment area, as well as with the team managers for each CMHT and discussed my interest in examining how clinicians initiated and designed requests for joint working during CMHT allocation meetings. Following this, I was invited to attend the CMHT allocation meetings, to meet the individual MDTs and to give a verbal presentation of the research and to share information packs and consent forms. The consent forms were then scrutinised by the team psychologist and by the researcher, to confirm that all team members had given consent. Teams were excluded if at least one clinician had refused to give consent. Three CMHTs agreed to take part in the research.

Data Generation

Five and half hours of naturalistic audio data was recorded from three allocation meetings from three CMHT teams. On average, 10 staff members were present during the meetings and approximately 233 individual cases were discussed. Audio data was initially transcribed orthographically.

In total, 35 extracts relating to requests for joint working were identified. This collection was assembled through repeatedly listening to the audio segments. The 35 extracts in the collection were then transcribed in line with the conventions outlined by Gail Jefferson (Lerner, 2004).

Findings

A principal finding from this analysis was the use of a stepwise progression into a request and the role of the chair in sanctioning or otherwise directing the outcome of the request. Our first example demonstrates a canonical way in which team members made a stepwise move into requesting. This stepwise move displayed the speaker's orientation to entitlement and contingency (Curl & Drew, 2008) thereby making explicit the obligation of another to comply (or not) with the request. In the following example, this obligation is built up by outlining a potential course of action using the modal verb "might".

Stepwise Progression into a Request

Extract 1: Team 2 at 30:50–31:46

(Key: TM = Team Manager; CMHN = Community Mental Health Nurse)

```
 1 TM      clearly but it's does she meet the
 2         [criteria for us]
 3 CMHN1   [↑yeah::      ] and that's what I've
 4         gotta sit down and do
 5         so ↑maybe what I ↑might do is invite somebody else
 6         to join me on that ↓appointment
 7 TM      [mm ]
 8 CMHN1   [jus'] so it's not just my thought processes
 9         it might be someone else >jus' to ↑kindov<
10         bounce it ↑off (.) and ↓clarify it
11         who did (.) met with (.)
12         did ↑you meet her with me=
13 CMHN2   =I think so yeah I'll come again
14 CMHN1   ↓yeah
```

At the start of this extract, the team manager, who is chairing the meeting, ascertains whether a particular service user is a suitable case for their consideration through clarifying whether the client meets the criteria. Once it has been established that a case falls within the remit of the team, the next step is normally to determine what course of action is required. The nurse (CMHN1) orientates to being selected to respond to this case and initially simply acknowledges that the issue of service criteria has been raised by the chair. The nurse then clarifies that they intend to carry out an assessment in order to determine whether the service user does match the criteria for consideration by the team. The nurse then embarks on a stepwise move into a request for another member of the team to work jointly with them during the assessment.

Rather than initially making a direct request for assistance, the nurse proposes a hypothetical course of action starting with the discourse marker "maybe" then using the modal verb "might" and the pro-term "somebody". This possible course of action clearly implicates others although which other, or others, is not specified. This potential course of action is acknowledged by the chair (line 7: "mm") though this minimal acknowledgement does not affiliate with the proposal. The nurse then embarks on an account which gives the reason for this course of action. It is noticeable how this account foregrounds the need of the nurse to have a second opinion rather than explaining the complexity of the case. Moreover, the requirements on the other are minimised through the use of the word "just" (line 9), thus reducing the implied amount of work required from other team members to conduct a joint appointment. Within the schema proposed by Curl and Drew, this account of the amount of work required is an orientation to the contingency of the request in progress. Having minimised the amount of work required, the nurse then moves into a direct request for the help of another member of the team. The nurse identifies a specific member of the team through an interrogatively formatted request ("did you meet her with me") which is valenced towards agreement. This format selects a specific other member of the team and given the prior hypothetical proposed course of action, it clearly carries the implication that this other member of the team has an obligation to help having previously done joint work with the nurse.

Making explicit this obligation orients to the entitlement of the nurse to make the request to this specific member of the team.

The next turn by the second nurse confirms that they have heard the prior turn as a request; not only does the team member confirm that they have met with the service user along with the first nurse ("I think so yeah"), they also immediately confirm that they will comply with the request and accompany the first nurse in the joint assessment. The first CMHN then takes up the offer for the joint appointment through the affiliative "yeah" before the team proceeds to discuss the specifics about arranging the appointment.

This request is developed through a stepwise sequence, namely a possible course of action (modal verb plus general pro-term), account for the course of action and interrogatively formatted direct request. The initial steps seem to lay the ground for moving into a request directed at a specific recipient. The directed request is made through an interrogative format valenced towards affirmative as a responsive second. In the corpus as a whole, this stepwise design of requests initiated with some-one/somebody as pro-terms plus the modal "might" was generally successful in eliciting compliance with requests.

Chair's Role in Directing the Outcome of Requests

One of the distinctive aspects of MDTs allocation meetings is that they are oriented to by the participants as meetings; that is, the design of turns and the sorts of actions in which they engage in enable members to constitute these encounters as meetings on a turn-by-turn basis (see Chapter 4). One of the particular features of "meeting talk" is the sorts of actions that the chairs of the meetings are entitled to take. One finding of this project concerned the role of the chair following requests. Normatively, it was the chair who made the response to the request particularly where the request did not specify that another member of the team was obliged to respond to the request directly (cf. Extract 1).

Extract 2: Team 3 at 1:02:32–1:03:12

(Key: CPSY = Clinical Psychologist; TM = Team Manager)

```
 1 CPSY      (.)↑can I do (.) a err an appointment >with a

 2           member< of the [↑team erm]=

 3 TM                        [°yeah°   ]

 4 CPSY      =for him (.) errm

 5           shall I just try an grab someone at random↓

 6           to find a time to [do   ]

 7 TM                          [↑send] an email with days

 8           and [times and I'll]

 9 CPSY          [yeah   erm   ]

10 TM          send the days and times I'll email around and

11           see what we can get

12 CPSY      .hh Tuesday or Wednesday ↑mo:rning or Monday

13           afternoon if anyone's available

14           (1.5)

15 TM        °okay°

16           (3.0)
```

This extract opens with the clinical psychologist requesting support through having an appointment with a service user along with another member of the team. It is delivered as an interrogative and in this format suggests that the psychologist has both the entitlement to request such an appointment, possibly through their expertise, and that there is an obligation on the team members to support this request in order to share the accountability. The team manager as chair acknowledges this request and by using the affirmative affiliates with it as legitimate. The psychologist then proposes a course of action using a similar design to that seen in Extract 1, specifically a modal verb ("shall") and pro-term ("someone"). The proposed course of action is also minimised through using "just" and suggesting that the person who can help is simply whoever is available ("grab someone at random") rather than a clinician with particular skills. This suggested course of action is geared towards confirmation as the second pair part. There is overlap by the chair, who interrupts before the next TRP has occurred (lines 6–7), as it is done in overlap, it is then repaired at line 10 with essentially a restatement of their prior turn. This interruption defeases the proposed course of action by identifying an alternative using the much stronger imperative form (lines 7–8, 10). This alternative course of action is also noticeable in that it does not implicate anyone else from the team as being obligated to fulfil the request.

In this extract, there is a direct request which is pursued through a proposed course of action. This proposed course of action is responded to by the chair who in turn resists and proposes an alternative less obligatory course of action. The chair's proposal is acknowledged by the psychologist, and this alternative course of action is pursued by the psychologist by offering days and times for an appointment. This pursuit is completed by a conditional which is now negatively valenced ("if anyone's available"). The response to this is a lapse (1.5 secs of silence) during which no member of the team confirms their availability at these times. There is a final acknowledgement by the chair which effectively closes this agenda item.

A further example of the chair proposing a course of action which resists a request for support is evident in the following extract. This extract follows a discussion where the Clinical Psychologist has described a service user who may benefit from engaging with a different member of the team following an initial assessment.

Extract 3: Team 1 (1:11:15–1:13:00)

(CPSY = Clinical Psychologist; TM = Team Manager)

```
1  CPSY    so it was really to bring her back to >think about
2          ↑really(.) cauz (1.0) .hh I don't feel it's
3          something for me to pick up just to do self-esteem
4          work
           (several lines omitted)
5  CPSY    so .hh I'm gonna call her back in but I wan'ed to
6          speak to the team ↑first, .hh before cu-so I could
7          actually ↑give her err eh-an idea ov' what we were
8          gonna offer
9  TM      ↑perha:ps err (.) I don't know I .hh thinking out
10         loud buh .hh it sounds like >there might some
11         signpostin'<(.) required around (.) her needs
12         as well
13 CPSY    hmm
```

Extract 3 shows how the Clinical Psychologist provides a problem-based justification, prior to initiating the request to "speak to the team first". This is communicated through the use of the preface ("so it was really to bring her back to think about") in line 1 and the long pause in line 2 which indicates that the subsequent talk is delicate (Silverman & Perakyla, 1990). This is followed by the upshot (Antaki, Barnes, & Leudar, 2005) in lines 2–3 ("I don't feel it's something for me to pick up"). The inference which this part of the turn makes available is that the proposed work with the service user is not within this psychologist's remit; indeed, the term "just" suggests that this work may not specifically require intervention from the psychologist. Making this inference available in turn suggests that this work may be undertaken by another clinician. This essentially primes the other speakers for the request that follows in lines 5–8. The request in lines 6–7 is identified through the rising intonation in lines 6 ("first") and 7 ("give") (Stivers & Rossano, 2010).

The Clinical Psychologist also shifts the accountability for actioning work with this service user to the other members of the MDT through use of the collective pronoun (line 7: "what we are gonna offer"). This is responded to with a suggestion for "signposting". The move to suggesting signposting is done through a turn which has the characteristics of a dispreferred turn shape. It is marked by a discourse marker (perhaps), palliatives (I don't know, thinking out loud), hesitancy and downgraded proposals (it sounds like) (lines 9–12). In this extract, there is a move to shifting the responsibility for this service user to the team as a whole. This move is resisted by the team manager with the suggestion of signposting. The team manager is also acting as chair of this meeting and through their resistance and suggestion of signposting abrogates the responsibility for other members of the team to take this work on. This displays the entitlements that are attendant on those who hold the chair's position to influence the course of decision-making.

Recommendations for Interprofessional Working

Many mental health services across the UK are experiencing pressures to manage high caseloads of service users with complex needs within the community. Consequently, clinicians may experience fewer opportunities for joint working, with many professionals lone working in the community. A joint working approach is beneficial as it enables clinicians to share accountability with other members of the MDT (Onyett, 2002). Joint working has been identified as having benefits not only for service users but also for clinicians (see Chapter 1). Joint working potentially brings the team together, at a time when practitioners may be feeling isolated, and provided them an opportunity to feel supported and to offer each other support (see Chapter 6).

It is important that clinicians consider how they can elicit the support of colleagues sensitively and delicately, particularly when services are facing pressures to offer services with fewer resources. It is also important for the chairs of MDT meetings to consider how they deal with requests from colleagues. In the two of the examples here, the chair resisted the request being made by the MDT member and the course of action proposed by the member was not ultimately agreed to. Where a request was successful it bypassed the chair and was directed to a specific member of the MDT. It should be incumbent on chairs to provide a clearer way forward following requests in order ensure that the team members retain a sense of efficacy and feel supported in their work.

A further suggestion is that clinicians should be encouraged to influence organisational change, through clear lines of communication between senior management and front-line clinicians, in order to contain concerns about gaps in service provision and to promote a sense of security that the issues are being addressed. This should take place in forums (e.g. clinical governance and operational meetings) that are attended by senior managers within the organisation, as this could inform the development of an action plan to address the issues being faced. For example, increased awareness of staffing vacancies could lead to an increase in budgets allocated to service and the advertisement and recruitment of new staff, as well as an increased focus on staff retention. This would inform better practices around leadership within organisations, as better communication would provide a supportive and conducive work environment for clinicians, thus enabling them to thrive within their roles (Onyett, 2002). This is noteworthy as it highlights the difficulties that clinicians may experience with regard to speaking out against decisions around the allocation of resources, particularly within services that are traditionally under-resourced, and the impact that these decisions have on service users.

Summary

This chapter offers guidance for mental health care professionals working within areas that are traditionally under-resourced such as CMHTs. The main focus has been on how clinicians articulate and enlist the support of others, through joint working, during times of limited resources. It is envisaged that through exploring the different designs and responses to requests, clinicians will be able to effectively communicate their needs for assistance and escalate their concerns where there are gaps in service provision, whilst also showing compassion to other members of the MDT.

Acknowledgements I would like to thank the clinicians and managers within the CMHTs that took part in this research. I would also like to thank the Adult Mental Health Psychology Team, in particular the Lead CMHT Psychologist, Dr Helen Brotherton, for their support throughout this project.

References

Antaki, C., Barnes, R., & Leudar, I. (2005). Self-disclosure as a situated interactional practice. *British Journal of Social Psychology, 44*(2), 181–199. https://doi.org/10.1348/014466604x15733.

Butler, J. (2005). Monitoring community mental health team caseloads: A systematic audit of practitioner caseloads using a criterion-based audit tool. *Advancing Practice in Bedfordshire, 2*(3), 95–105.

Curl, T. S., & Drew, P. (2008). Contingency and action: A comparison of two forms of requesting. *Research on Language & Social Interaction, 41*(2), 129–153. https://doi.org/10.1080/08351810802028613.

Department of Health. (2002) *Mental health policy implementation guide: Community mental health teams*. London: DoH.

Fox, B. (2015). On the notion of pre-request. *Discourse Studies, 17*(1), 41–63. https://doi.org/10.1177/1461445614557762.

Griffiths, L. (2001). Categorising to exclude: The discursive construction of cases in community mental health teams. *Sociology of Health & Illness, 23*(5), 678–700. https://doi.org/10.1111/1467-9566.00271.

Heritage, J., & Clayman, S. (2010). *Talk in action: Interactions, identities, and institutions*. Oxford: Wiley.

Independent Mental Health Taskforce to NHS England. (2016). *The five year forward view for mental health*. Retrieved from https://www.england.nhs.uk/wp-content/uploads/2016/02/Mental-Health-Taskforce-FYFV-final.pdf. Accessed on 28 June 2018.

Kendrick, K. H., & Drew, P. (2016). Recruitment: Offers, requests, and the organization of assistance in interaction. *Research on Language and Social Interaction, 49*(1), 1–19. https://doi.org/10.1080/08351813.2016.1126436.

Lerner, G. H. (Ed.). (2004). *Conversation analysis*. Philadelphia: John Benjamins.

Onyett, S. (2002). *Teamworking in mental health*. Basingstoke: Palgrave Macmillan.

Sands, N. (2009). An exploration of clinical decision making in mental health triage. *Archives of Psychiatric Nursing, 23*(4), 298–308. https://doi.org/10.1016/j.apnu.2008.08.002.

Schegloff, E. A. (2006). *Sequence organization in interaction: A primer in conversation analysis*. Cambridge: Cambridge University Press.

Silverman, D., & Perakyla, A. (1990). AIDS counselling: The interactional organisation of talk about "delicate" issues. *Sociology of Health & Illness, 12*(3), 293–318. https://doi.org/10.1111/1467-9566.ep11347251.

Stivers, T., & Rossano, F. (2010). Mobilizing response. *Research on Language & Social Interaction, 43*(1), 3–31. https://doi.org/10.1080/08351810903471258.

West, M. A. (1994). *Effective teamwork*. Leicester: British Psychological Society.

Zinken, J., & Rossi, G. (2016). Assistance and other forms of cooperative engagement. *Research on Language and Social Interaction, 49*(1), 20–26. https://doi.org/10.1080/08351813.2016.1126439.

10

Sharing Information and Retelling Stories in a Memory Clinic MDT Meeting

Jennifer Dickenson and Cordet Smart

Introduction

This chapter focuses upon the interactions between clinicians within a UK based memory clinic. Memory clinics are widely used across the UK to facilitate the process of identifying and diagnosing dementia. To receive a diagnosis of dementia, a decline in one or more of these areas needs to be identified: learning and memory; language; executive function; complex attention; and perceptual-motor or social cognition. The decline also needs to cause significant impairment in social or occupational functioning and represent a significant decline from a previous level of functioning (American Psychiatric Association, 2013).

J. Dickenson (✉)
Devon Partnership NHS Trust, Exeter, UK
e-mail: jenniferdickenson@nhs.net

C. Smart
School of Psychology, University of Plymouth, Plymouth, UK
e-mail: cordet.smart@plymouth.ac.uk

© The Author(s) 2018
C. Smart and T. Auburn (eds.), *Interprofessional Care and Mental Health*,
The Language of Mental Health, https://doi.org/10.1007/978-3-319-98228-1_10

Multidisciplinary team (MDT) memory clinics are recommended to contribute to effective assessments, earlier diagnosis and interventions (All-Party Parliamentary Group on Dementia, 2012; DoH, 2012; Wolfs, Kessels, Dirksen, Severens, & Verheij, 2008). UK national guidelines suggest that MDT working within memory clinics should consist of 'A medical practitioner and a multidisciplinary team consisting of at least two other professions' (The Royal College of Psychiatrists, 2014, p. 9). This allows for knowledge, skills and expertise across different disciplines to be shared, promoting a biopsychosocial approach (NHS England, 2014). Incorporating this model means the biological factors can be considered alongside the psychological and social factors. This provides a holistic understanding of the service user's difficulties, which can help identify the most suitable outcomes for the service user and their supporters (Specter & Orrell, 2010).

MDT working within the NHS is highly recommended; however, there is currently little research into how MDTs interact and communicate within different services offered within the NHS. This book provides detailed examples of MDT working within different settings within the healthcare services and this chapter examines how information is shared between clinicians within a memory clinic diagnostic meeting.

A particular concern in memory clinics is that people with dementia often have very specific challenges in communication. Nilsson, Ekström, and Majlesi (2018) summarise some of the known challenges, including showing how people with dementia or memory difficulties can frequently experience feeling left out from conversations. Their supporters or family members often have to learn to speak for them, which can ensure that their voice is heard and represented, but can also be problematic in terms of how the person with memory difficulties is themselves represented. The memory clinic introduces a further layer of difficulty, as the experiences of the person with memory difficulties must be further translated by clinicians; thus, it is these effects that are the focus of this chapter.

Project Overview

The project focused on a typical UK memory clinic. In these clinics, one clinician meets with the service users (often an assistant psychologist), another meets with their supporter[1] (often a support worker or mental health nurse) and a third (normally the psychiatrist or the geriatrician) reviews brain scans and medication. They then meet to share information with their colleagues to develop a diagnosis, before the lead clinician, usually the psychiatrist, provides feedback to the service user and supporter. The representation of the views of service users and supporters is therefore important to the development of the diagnosis.

To examine how service user and supporter perspectives were displayed, we drew on CA understandings of storytelling. Other interactional research cites storytelling as a key practice in delivering information about service users and their families in absentia (Mandelbaum, 2014). A study examining nursing shift handovers found that when a clinician was retelling an event, or storytelling, they would use reported speech to help make sense of non-routine measures (Bangerter, Mayor, & Pekarek Doehler, 2011). In reported speech, one purports to use the exact words of a speaker, whereas in indirect reported speech the speaker's words are adapted to the current circumstances (Holt & Clift, 2007). Reported speech appears to have the action of 'showing' rather than 'telling' (Holt, 2000) and enables a speaker to convey an evaluation of the information shared within the story (Holt, 2000; Holt & Clift, 2007; Sidnell, 2006). Thus within the memory clinic, it might be useful to understand how this evaluation affected the way that the service user and supporters' difficulties are discussed. Further, specific to the experience of dementia, there is a question about how the possible changes in memory of a service user are represented within this storytelling, and how their story might ultimately be treated differently within a diagnostic discussion.

---

[1]"Supporter" is used to refer to family members, friend or carer.

When retelling information or storytelling, people are said to use different domains of knowledge to make claims to the credibility of the information that they present, this is known as epistemics. This can also be related to power dynamics within an interaction and is discussed further in Chapter 5. The clinicians professional 'role' can be considered as their status, assigned outside of the interaction, but within the meeting people have the ability to present a particular epistemic stance, depending on how they design their speech (Heritage, 2012). This chapter aims to support the development of communication practices between clinicians that can facilitate the implementation of a biopsychosocial approach to the assessment of dementia. Specific objectives were to identify and analyse interactional practices used by assistant psychologists and support workers that were able to represent the perspective of the service user and their supporters.

Method

The data within this chapter were collected from one memory clinic within the UK. Six clinicians (2 psychiatrists; 1 assistant psychologist, 2 support workers and 1 mental health nurse) were present on data recording days. Informed consent was gained from all clinicians. The data were collected on 7 separate days, during which 21 MDT diagnostic discussion meetings were video recorded. The meetings ranged between 06:42 minutes and 37:58 minutes.

The meetings generally consisted of the support worker speaking first, relaying the information from their assessment with the supporter, then the assistant psychologist sharing the information from their assessment with service user and finally the psychiatrist asking questions. Following the meeting the psychiatrist would provide feedback to the service user and their supporter.

Conversation analysis was used to analyse the data (Drew & Heritage, 1992; Sidnell & Stivers, 2014; as discussed in Chapter 2). Identifiable information was deleted, and pseudonyms of names and places were used in transcripts. All data were transcribed orthographically. Transcripts were then reviewed to identify practices where the assistant psychologist or support worker represented the experiences of the service user and supporter. Jeffersonian transcription (Jefferson, 2004) was then used and the practices were interrogated using conversation analysis.

Credibility of analysis was enhanced through regular presentation and discussion at CARP (Conversation Analytic Research at Plymouth, https://www.plymouth.ac.uk/research/psychology/conversation-ana-lytic-research-group) throughout the project to check interpretation of extracts. In addition, joint analysis (see Chapter 14) was conducted with two of the participants to promote researcher and participant collaboration. This informed the analysis stage; provided a reflective space for the participants to talk about their experiences of working within a memory clinic; and helped identify patterns of interaction. Feedback on the analytic focus of storytelling was also gained; for example, the assistant psychologist commented that they would retell particular stories during the MDT meeting based upon their sense of the service user and their assumption about the cause of memory problems. They also suggested that this may cause a 'bias' during the MDT diagnostic discussion.

Analysis

Storytelling emerged as a key practice used to report on assessments of both the service user and supporters; 185 occurrences of storytelling were identified. We were interested in the differences between how the supporter assessors and the service user assessor's reported within the MDT meeting with the psychiatrist, particularly as there may be some question over what the service user reportedly said, depending on their level of memory function. These constituted three different practices, how the:

1. Supporter assessors used retelling of stories told to them by the supporter about their lives (96 occurrences);
2. Service user assessors used retellings of stories told to them by the service user about their lives (36 occurrences); and
3. Service user assessors retold stories of their interaction with the service user during the assessment (53 occurrences).

Each practice is discussed in turn, and the implications this has for a diagnostic meeting about dementia. Notably, the supporter assessors retold stories told to them, but did not tell stories of the interaction. Stories of the interaction were used by service user assessors and seemed to be used to question the veracity of the reported stories of service users.

Supporter Assessors Retelling Stories Told to Them by the Supporter About Their Lives

Tellings by supporter assessors used frequent direct reported speech to 'voice' the family within the MDTs. This is exemplified in Extract 1, where the team is discussing the service user's abilities in terms of new learning. This includes drawing on cognitive skills including executive functioning and memory domains.

Extract 1: Indirect Reported Speech and Claim to Knowledge

Key: CP: consultant psychiatrist; SW: support worker; AP: assistant psychologist

```
1   CP:  <so lear:ning a new gadget is a   bit worse↑>
2   SW:  yeah he said th-the-the children >were trying to teach her
3        to use< an an iPad and sort of (.) you know social me:dia
4        stuff but she's not interested in it so it's just like we:ll↑
5   CP:  ◦okay◦
6   SW:  >I'd rather be< playin up↑ with my pla:n[ts]◦
7   CP:                                          [mmm]
8   SW:  [you kno(hhh)w] huhuhuh
9   CP:  [mmm mmm]              ◦true true◦
```

The topic of learning new things is introduced by the psychiatrist in line 1, who provides an upshot formulation: 'so learning a new gadget is a bit worse', with an upward intonation on the 'worse' appearing to invite confirmation. The supporter assessor then accesses an epistemic domain unavailable to either the service user assessor or the psychiatrist, that is, what was said to the supporter assessor. In line 2, she says 'yeah, he said…'. She is the only one who knows what he did say, and so cannot be questioned by either of the other clinicians, giving her credibility. Having taken the floor, she then continues through what might be described as a 'stepwise transition' (Jefferson, 2004) into talking as if she were a supporter (Holt, 2000). In line 4, she states 'she's (the service user is) not interested in it…' as if she (the supporter assessor) herself knows what the service user might be interested in, yet this is outside of her epistemic territory as she has had no direct experience of the service user. Telling the story as if she was a supporter or family member seemed to provide a 'pseudo'-epistemic claim. Finally, in line 7 she makes a statement as if she were the service user 'I'd rather be playing with my plants'.

During the joint analysis session, the supporter assessor stated that when she retells an account during the meeting she 'wants to get it right' and so 'tries to retell it the same way it was told' to her, suggesting that the support worker is also intending to advocate for the supporter. The current analysis suggests that this is not only about displaying a 'representation of truth', but also can be highly persuasive in gaining the floor, as others present in the room don't have access to the same remembered events.

Service User Assessor Retelling Stories: Where a Service User Is Displayed as Having Insight

The service user assessor applied two main strategies—retelling the service user's perspective (36 extracts identified) and telling the story of his interaction with the service user (53 extracts identified). Within the first practice, of telling the story of the service user, both direct reported speech and indirect reported speech were used, but when the information being gathered during the assessment appeared to show inconsistencies, the service user assessor would juxtapose together the information to form an inference. This is illustrated in Extract 2.

Extract 2: Retelling the Story of the Client and Highlighting Inconsistencies

Key: CP: consultant psychiatrist; SW: support worker; AP: assistant psychologist

```
1   AP:  >he said about forgetting< what's on T:V when he walks out
2        the room so he's watched something he walks out=
3   SW:  =°can't[remember what it is°]
4   AP:        [and then he's like] (.) oh >what was on< you know
5        and he's already >forgotten< erm he wasn't able to recall
6        what he had to eat like I said he was able to recall (.)a
7        bit about the n:ews=
8   CP:  =mmm
9   AP:  >basically<
10  SW:  [·hhh huhuh]
```

Extract 2 is located 7 minutes into a 13-minute diagnostic meeting: the supporter assessor had already provided feedback from their assessment. The assistant psychologist had been speaking for two minutes and informed his colleagues that the service user scored low on the cognitive assessment which would be indicative of a dementia diagnosis. On line 1, the assistant psychologist used indirect reported speech, introduced with 'he said' to retell a story told to him by the service user about his experiences of forgetting. In this description, the service user assessor was able to draw attention to an experience that the service user had been able to present—forgetting what was on the television. These forms of assessment appeared designed for this particular context of memory assessment. They were normatively received with displays of affiliation from other professionals. For example, here, the supporter assessor pre-empts the service user assessor's formulation, stating that the service user 'can't remember' in line 3. The two reporting speakers, the supporter assessor and the service user assessor, therefore already conjointly display clinical formulating in their reporting of findings. The service user assessor's use of direct reported speech in line 4 'oh what was on' then seems to display credibility for the clinical formulation that they are developing regarding the service users' reduced memory abilities.

Service User Assessor Retelling Stories: Where the Insight of a Service User Might Be Questioned

Representing the service user's perspective was more complex than representation of family experiences, due to the question of credibility around the service user's cognitive abilities. The service user assessor had to accomplish the complex work of representing the service user's perspective in a valuing manner and questioning it at the same time. This seemed to present an ethical struggle for the service user assessor, evident in the particularly delicate manner in which they represented their assessments. To negotiate this dilemma, the service user assessor appeared to engage in a drawn-out practice where they would first retell not only the story of the service user, but also of their own interaction with them within the room, demonstrating inconsistency or discrepancy in information (which we term the 'description' phase of the practice). The service user assessor would then use an 'upshot' followed by an explicit 'clinical formulation'. This practice seemed to enable implicit concerns to be raised, relating to the service user's level of insight. This is exemplified in Extract 3.

Extract 3 is located at 7 minutes within an MDT diagnostic meeting which lasted 20 minutes. The supporter assessor had provided a summary of the information gathered from the service user's husband. The service user assessor had been speaking for three minutes. The extract is divided into two sections to illustrate how the different devices within talk were applied during the sequence: Extract 3a 'Description' and Extract 3b 'Upshot' and 'Clinical Formulation'.

Extract 3a: The Service User Assessor's Description Demonstrating Implicit Uncertainty
Key: CP: consultant psychiatrist; SW: support worker; AP: assistant psychologist

```
 1   AP:  ·tt err ADL:s you've cov:ered the:re so th -th:e <finances
 2        were> ok:ay th-the husband generally is doing it >but
 3        then she will do the odd< statement >·she hasn't had any
 4        problems ·< (.)> that's because it sounds like they manage
→5        it together·< ·hhh erm PIN >seems okay< she said oh oh I
 6        have to think and have it written down >I don't use it
 7        very often<
 8   CP:  mmmm
→9   AP:  but then I said(.)you know in respect to shopping >you
10        know when you go to the shops <
→11  CP:  mmhmm
12   AP:  do you pay by cash then↑ she said oh no I pay by ca:rd
13        and then (.) I said how are you at remembering that code
14        >oh oh that's fine< so it doesn't
```

Extract 3a illustrates the 'description' phase of this sequence that was used, where the insight of the service user is made questionable. In this phase, 3 particular features are notable: (1) the intensity or the experiences that are presented; (2) the presentation of inconsistency; and (3) the way that an overt diagnostic claim was mitigated. Firstly, the scene is set for this practice with a detailed description of finances in lines 1–5. Edwards and Potter (1993) suggest that these detailed accounts can give credence to a subsequent claim. The presentation of inconsistency is achieved with considerable delicacy between lines 5 and 15. In line 5, the service user assessor states: 'PIN seems OK' and then uses direct reported speech: 'have it written down' to support his claim that the service user can remember their PIN number. However, in line 9, the service user assessor initiates a contrastive position, suggesting an inconsistency: 'but then I said…', and in this instance, the reported speech appears to have the action of demonstrating the inconsistency rather than explicitly stating it. This contrast structure appears to display a position of 'reduced personal responsibility' for the service user assessor, as he reports two misaligned events, which demonstrate inconsistency, so his responsibility for this interpretation is removed. This approach might also demonstrate that this inconsistency is a sensitive issue (Goffman, 1981). The described information is receipted by the psychiatrist with minimal acknowledgement tokens in lines 8 and 11, 'mmm' (line 8) and 'mmhmm' (line 11). In lines 12–13, the service user assessor again reports the service user's speech where the service user suggests that there is no problem with use of her card, conflicting with the earlier statement that she has to write it down.

The service user assessor, then, appears to mitigate any diagnostic claim that they might be making, through the use of reported speech and use of a range of tentative prefaces. In this way, through the retelling of the interaction, the service user assessor is able to present the situation as a 'truth' which is less affected by their personal assessment. This appears to be a way of managing the boundaries of their role as a more junior member of staff than the psychiatrist, but also managing the stage of the meeting as the concluding 'diagnostic' part has not yet been reached. For example, on line 4 he used the preface 'it sounds like', rather than a declarative statement or imperative term such as 'it is'. This also occurred on line 5 when he prefaces 'okay' with 'seems'.

Following the descriptive stage of the sequence, the service user assessor provided a summary and clinical formulation which is illustrated in Extract 3b.

Extract 3b: The Assistant Psychologist's Implicit Uncertainty Upshot and Formulation
Key: CP: consultant psychiatrist; SW: support worker; AP: assistant psychologist

```
    11   AP:    do you pay by cash then↑ she said oh no I pay by ca:rd

    12          and then (.) I said how are you at remembering that

➡  13          code >oh oh that's fine< so it doesn't

    14   SW:    [Ah yeah I see]

    15   CP:    [(yes sure) ]

➡  16   AP:    doesn't seem like she does have any problems with the

    17          ones she >uses regularly< erm
```

The service user assessor continues the story in lines 11–13 to reach an upshot contrastive statement in line 13: 'so it doesn't', which is again left unfinished—it is not yet the time to formulate a diagnosis. This appeared to have several functions, to inform the listeners that he had observed something contrastive; state his position in regard to the claim; and invite either agreement or disagreement from the supporter assessor and psychiatrist. This was instantly recognised by both clinicians and they respond 'ah I see' on line 14 and 'yes sure' on line 15. These affiliative responses seem to provide the service user assessor with increased confidence to display a clinical formulation. He summarises in line 16: 'it doesn't seem like she does have any problems with the ones that she uses regularly' (lines 16 and 17). Through retelling the interaction, the service user assessor appeared to establish an epistemic territory, increasing his credibility and enabling him to question the service user's that she had difficulties with memory in terms of managing money.

Summary

This chapter highlights that there is currently limited research into how different professionals work together within a memory clinic to share assessment information during an MDT diagnostic meeting. Making a decision about a diagnosis of dementia is a complex process which consists of drawing upon multiple pieces of information, and here we focused on how the psychological and social experiences were reported in the implementation of a biopsychosocial approach.

The analysis revealed that clinicians adopt different storytelling practices to help share assessment information. Clinicians may use these interactional practices unintentionally. However, it appears that these devices have specific functions, such as, demonstrating a sensitive issue including a discrepancy in information in the case of assessing the service user. The different devices of retelling the experiences of service users and their supporters and retelling stories of interactions from the assessment appear to have an underlying persuasive function which can help to seek affiliation and agreement between the clinicians within the MDT diagnostic meeting. These different approaches seem to reflect the ways that family members have been found in other settings to interact with their relatives with memory difficulties—that is, where having a memory difficulty gives rise to greater talk about the person, rather than just relying on what they report. This may of course be part of clinical discussion—it is necessary to talk about a person in order to come to a formulation of what is of concern for them. However, the specific approach, focusing on inconsistencies, is perhaps most salient for this context and might be examined in the context of reflecting on how service users might experience this.

The particular challenges of the meeting moving through a 'process' of different stages (reporting and formulating), and memory difficulties not necessarily being objectively observable, seems to particularly lend itself to 'demonstrations'. 'Demonstrations' and retelling of stories enables for further consideration of how memory might be compromised and identifies conflicts between what has been reported and what is observed.

Implications for Interprofessional Working

- Reflecting on the diagnostic discussion and how claims are made might be important—as reports are not given without 'bias'.
- It may be easier to report on memory difficulties than non-memory difficulties—we say here that memory problems were the first interpretation.

- It might be relevant to continue to consider how the person with dementia feels, and whether these assessments sometimes 'leave out' their experiences, due to the difficulty ascertaining and reporting them.
- An inviting approach that highlights discrepancies rather than stating an assumed diagnosis may serve to encourage a more collaborative approach to MDT working (Stivers, 2008).

Acknowledgements We would like to thank all the staff from the memory clinic service for their support in conducting this study. We would also like to especially thank the clinicians who agreed to participate.

References

All-Party Parliamentary Group on Dementia. (2012). *Unlocking diagnosis: The key to improving the lives of people with dementia*. London: House of Commons.

American Psychiatric Association. (2013). *Diagnostic and statistical manual of mental disorders* (5th ed.). Washington, DC: Author.

Bangerter, A., Mayor, E., & Pekarek Doehler, S. (2011). Reported speech in conversational storytelling during nursing shift handover meetings. *Discourse Processes, 48*(3), 183–214. https://doi.org/10.1080/0163853X.2010.519765.

Department of Health (DoH). (2012). *Prime Minister's challenge on dementia—Delivering major improvements in dementia care and research by 2015*. DoH: London.

Drew, P., & Heritage, J. (1992). Analyzing talk at work: An introduction. In P. Drew & J. Heritage (Eds.), *Talk at work: Interaction in institutional settings* (pp. 3–65). Cambridge: Cambridge University Press.

Edwards, D., & Potter, D. (1993). *Discursive psychology*. London: Sage.

Goffman, E. (1981). *Forms of talk*. Philadelphia: University of Pennsylvania Press.

Heritage, J. (2012). Epistemics in action: Action formation and territories of knowledge. *Research on Language and Social Interaction, 45*(1), 1–29. https://doi.org/10.1080/08351813.2012.646684.

Holt, E. (2000). Reporting and reacting: Concurrent responses to reported speech. *Research on Language and Social Interaction, 33*(4), 425–454. https://doi.org/10.1207/S15327973RLSI3304_04.

Holt, E., & Clift, R. (2007). *Reporting talk: Reported speech in interaction. Studies in interactional sociolinguistics.* Cambridge: Cambridge University Press.

Jefferson, G. (2004). Glossary of transcript symbols with an introduction. *Pragmatics and Beyond New Series, 125,* 13–34.

Mandelbaum, J. (2014). Storytelling in conversation. In J. Sidnell & T. Stivers (Eds.), *The handbook of conversational analysis* (pp. 350–369). Chichester: Wiley.

National Health Service (NHS) England. (2014). *MDT Development— Working towards an effective multidisciplinary/multiagency team.* Retrieved from https://www.england.nhs.uk/wp-content/uploads/2015/01/mdt-dev-guid-flat-fin.pdf.

Nilsson, E., Ekström, A., Majlesi, A. R. (2018). Speaking for and about a spouse with dementia: A matter of inclusion or exclusion? *Discourse Studies,* 1–22. https://doi.org/10.1177/1461445618770482.

The Royal College of Psychiatrists. (2014). *Memory services national accreditation programme (MSNAP)* (4th ed.). London: RCPsych.

Sidnell, J. (2006). Coordinating gesture, talk, and gaze in reenactments. *Research on Language and Social Interaction, 39*(4), 377–409. https://doi.org/10.1207/s15327973rlsi3904_2.

Sidnell, J., & Stivers, T. (2014). *The handbook of conversation analysis.* Chichester: Wiley.

Spector, A., & Orrell, M. (2010). Using a biopsychosocial model of dementia as a tool to guide clinical practice. *International Psychogeriatrics, 22*(6), 957–965. https://doi.org/10.1017/S1041610210000840.

Stivers, T. (2008). Stance, alignment, and affiliation during storytelling: When nodding is a token of affiliation. *Research on Language and Social Interaction, 41*(1), 31–57.

Wolfs, C. A. G., Kessels, A., Dirksen, C. D., Severens, J. L., & Verheij, F. R. J. (2008). Integrated multidisciplinary diagnostic approach for dementia care: Randomised controlled trial. *British Journal of Psychiatry, 192,* 300–305.

Part IV

Patient Centred Interactions in Team Meetings

11

Advocacy for Service Users and Carers in Community Learning Disability Team Meetings When Service Users and Carers Are Absent

Cordet Smart and Holly Reed

Introduction

In recent years, there has been a push to make health care more patient centred. The term patient-centred care covers numerous aspects of care (Gluyas, 2015), including the idea that healthcare professionals should share information, power and responsibility by engaging both service users and their family and/or carers in the care process, allowing service users to have more of a say regarding the nature of their care. A number of studies across different health-care settings have shown that patient-centred care is cost-effective, increases service user satisfaction and cuts the length of hospital stays (Hansson et al., 2015; Sklar, Aarons, O'Connell, Davidson, & Groessl, 2015; Stone, 2008). However, one of the challenges of

C. Smart (✉) · H. Reed (✉)
School of Psychology, University of Plymouth, Plymouth, UK
e-mail: cordet.smart@plymouth.ac.uk

H. Reed
e-mail: holly.reed@students.plymouth.ac.uk

© The Author(s) 2018
C. Smart and T. Auburn (eds.), *Interprofessional Care and Mental Health*,
The Language of Mental Health, https://doi.org/10.1007/978-3-319-98228-1_11

patient-centred care is the different interpretations that people have of what might be in a patient's best interests. Within a multidisciplinary team setting especially where the service user or their carer is absent, then promoting the interests of the service user falls upon the professional members of the team who have knowledge, directly or indirectly of that service user. We have suggested that the activity of promoting the interests of the service user within an MDT setting is a form of advocacy. Therefore, current chapter focuses on advocacy, and the different ways in which this is accomplished within multidisciplinary team meetings where the service user is absent. In this chapter, we focus on MDTs within Learning Disability services. The aim of the MDT meetings investigated here, was to decide what the service might be able to offer to those who had been referred to them.

One of the difficulties for those who wish to promote the interests of people living with Learning Disabilities is that such people have been found to be more susceptible to submissiveness, saying what they think others want to hear (Henry & Gudjonsson, 1999). Booth and Booth (1996) identified four areas of challenge when engaging with individuals with learning disabilities regarding what they want: inarticulateness and impaired language skills; unresponsiveness in open questioning; difficulties with generalising and thinking in abstract terms; and difficulty with time and problems with recall, impacting on their ability to tell their story. Research has shown that some attempts at patient-centred care do not always have the desired effects when targeted at individuals with learning disabilities. Pilnick, Clegg, Murphy, and Almack (2010) found that in trying to empower individuals with Learning Disabilities, complex questions were sometimes asked and if the individual with the Learning Disability did not respond with an answer viewed as appropriate by the professionals, decisions were often made for them, sometimes while they were not even in the room. In order not to miss key concerns for service users and their carers, teams have emphasised the importance of multidisciplinary assessment.

Recognition of the vulnerability of particular populations has led to the increased use of advocates within healthcare settings. In some cases, individuals are legally entitled to have an independent advocate (Mental

Health Act, 1983; Mental Capacity Act, 2005), receiving this from the NHS. However, many charities also provide advocacy services, such as Mind, Mencap (who cater exclusively to individuals with learning disabilities) and VoiceAbility. Mind define advocacy in health care as 'getting support from another person to help you express your views and wishes, and help you stand up for your rights'.

Advocacy can occur not just from individual sources, but is also a key consideration within MDTs, and it seems somewhat remiss to assume that healthcare professionals as part of their roles do not intend to act on behalf of the patient. In the USA, there is a new role emerging in MDT meetings where one staff member specifically acts as the patient advocate (Campagna, 2013). The need for this role, it is argued, is to ensure that a holistic perspective is maintained, and that sight is not lost of the experiences of individuals. This is particularly relevant when staff must also be mindful of the full stretch of the service and limited resources. Research by McGrath, Holewa, and McGrath (2006) found that the conflict between the medico-centrism of doctors and the personal knowledge held by nurses often causes nurses to feel the need to advocate for their service users. They found that professional and clinical confidence and experience were needed to successfully engage in the process of advocacy. Indeed, there are a number of papers suggesting that part of the nurse's role is to tell the story of service users. A central question then is how advocacy is accomplished within team meetings and what impact does such advocacy have on the formulation of the service user's care plan.

Project Overview

The research aim was to examine practices of advocacy in team meetings. The research protocol was the same as the main project as outlined in Chapters 3 and 4. That is, the study used a naturalistic design, recording and analysing direct conversation between healthcare professionals during multidisciplinary team meetings; meetings were recorded from Community Learning Disability Services.

Professionals in these teams included: clinical psychologists (including trainees); community nurses; assistant practitioners; learning disability nurses; psychiatrists; continuing healthcare nurses; occupational therapists and physiotherapists, although exactly who was present in the meetings was dependant on the type of meeting, the particular service and availability. In total, 27 hours of meeting talk was collected across four different sites. The recordings included six different types of meetings which the teams referred to as business meetings; allocation meetings; peer review meetings; professional meetings; diagnostic meetings and multidisciplinary meetings. Meetings were initially orthographically transcribed. Extracts constituting advocacy were identified and then transcribed using Jeffersonian conventions (1984) and analysed using Conversation Analysis. Exclusion and inclusion criteria for what constituted advocacy were generated in the research team and within CARP (Conversation Analysis Research at Plymouth), a data analysis and research group. Inclusion criteria were: descriptions of service users, their needs and a rationale for why this necessitated a decision. 71 excerpts were identified, which divided into four types of advocacy.

Analysis was undertaken individually by the first and second authors, and taken to a Conversation Analysis Group at Plymouth University. Participants engaged in joint-analysis sessions and follow up discussions in order to help establish the plausibility of the findings (see Chapter 14).

Findings

Advocacy occurs throughout the team meetings as service users are discussed, this study focused on occasions where clinicians presented a case to overcome barriers to meeting service user needs. These occurred in 3 main contexts:

1. where there was a gatekeeping issue concerning access to services, this tended to be an issue internal to the MDT;

2. where services external to the MDT were creating barriers to meeting the service users needs; and
3. where others within the social network of the service user (such as family) were creating barriers to meeting the service user's needs.

There were different ways in which these occasions of advocacy appeared within the meetings although all instances in our collection were constituted through forms of storytelling about a service user's life. This observation questions the assumption that advocacy can be considered as a single activity. We identified four different practices which were used by staff to advocate for service users and carers within story tellings: use of personal emotional responses, direct and indirect reported speech, re-enactments and contrast structures. All of these ways of constituting advocacy were designed to persuade the meeting to adopt a course of action helpful to the service user.

Advocacy Within the MDT: Use of Emotion and Indirect Reported Speech to Punctuate Life Stories

The substantive corpus of data included allocations meetings, where it is the role of clinicians to decide whether or not a service user will be accepted into the service. This role inevitably included some 'gatekeeping' for the service. In some cases, a speaker would discuss a service user as if they were likely to be turned down. Advocates then moved into storytelling in order to provide a compelling case for why the team might consider the service user as an exceptional case. The use of advocacy at these points is illustrated in Extract 1. The extract shows how the speaker engages in storytelling to account for the service user having need of support. There has been some confusion around whether this service user should access Adult Mental Health or Learning Disability services. This potential uncertainty appears to give rise to a storytelling example to elaborate on why this service user should be accepted.

Extract 1: Stories Using Emotion and Reported Speech
(JAN: Learning disability nurse; SAR: Chair)

```
1    JAN:   ye:ah she was told pr:eviously by a doctor (0.1) a long

2            time ago not >not with in this team< that er:m if she

3            took some medication the m↑:an would go away °because

4            she always sees the man↓=

5    SAR:   yeah

6    JAN:   =out the window↓ outside° >And then the man didn't

7            go away< when she took the medication s:o=

8    SAR:   [°I see° ]

9    JAN:   [=You know] so that created difficulties and sort of

10           hopelessness I think (.) but (.) erm (.) >but

11           her husband< seems to be a incredibly positive in her

12           life and er you know a really sort of good carer and

13           source of support for her

14   SAR:   hmm

15   JAN:   but it ju she just ye:ah it just worries me and >it

16           saddens me cause< this woman doesn't (0.2) she just

17           doesn't get any help but like she's ap↑pearing again

18           >you know what I mean< she she obviously needs

19           something from so:mebody >or has a need that's on

20           there< but she just doesn't get any help from anyone

21           really and then it just goes off

22           [like we'll probably get another referral in a]=

23   SAR:   [got a  feeling  there  is  like  some  engage=]

24   JAN    =years' time again

25   SAR:    =ment issues though she had been referred for some
```

```
26              kind of talking therapy and °didn't° re:ally engage
27    JAN:      °has she,°
28    SAR:      I think it I'd have to go over her [letters]
29    JAN:                                         [I think] she
30              doesn't engage (.) you know,
31    SAR:      ye:ah
32    JAN:      but but I think that rather than maybe attempt build
33              up that relationship (0.2) Sam makes people
34              discharge when she's (.) like not attending one
35              appointment or you know, but this is a
36              woman with clini- chronic mental health issues sh she
37              probably won't attend the first appointment
```

Prior to this turn, the team discuss that it is not clear whether the service user has a learning disability, and that the service user doesn't 'really fit' the team. Jan then elaborates on the 'history' in line 1. This could be considered as the launch and the background of the story (see Mandelbaum, 2015). She presents the general introduction that this occurred in the past, and also anonymises the comment 'not within this team' (line 2). Then, using indirect reported speech to highlight the difficulty 'if she took some medication the man would go away' (lines 5–6), and then the upshot in lines 8–9 that the man didn't go away. In all of our examples, we observed the use of reported speech either direct (exemplified later) or indirect as here, which as Holt (2017) comments, often comes at the 'peak' of a storytelling. Within these accounts, we then later see an emotional 'plea' in lines 17–19—'it just worries me' and it saddens me—this repetition seems to suggest that there is some form of moral position that there is a claim for services to help—a claim to a deontic position, but also an emotional, empathic concerns, 'it saddens me because this woman doesn't she just doesn't get any help'. This is a display of empathy towards the service user. The construction mirrors that seen by Hepburn and Potter (2007) in helplines. In helplines, Hepburn and Potter found that call takers reformulated the mental state of service users and its origins. Here, we see that Jan owns her own emotional responses, saying that she feels sad. She then formulates this as because of this lady not getting any help (line 19), which is subsequently repeated. This then moves to the upshot for the team meeting in lines 21–23 'she obviously needs something from somebody'. There is then some resistance in the team—line 34, 'she doesn't engage (.) you know'. This is countered by the suggestion that there needs to be more attempt to engage—and a normalising that where people might have chronic mental health difficulties this would be an expectation, which she is able to claim, based on the story provided. In this way, advocacy includes accounting for why it is difficult for this particular service user to engage. The story provides a historical account, which we often see as more difficult to overcome (see also examples in Chapter 5). It seems to enable a reopening of the case by suggesting that the initial difficulty lay with engagement with services, and therefore services 'ought' now to offer support for this service user. Griffiths and Hughes (1994) have shown that in allocating services, choices are sometimes made by taking into account the deservedness of the individual in question. There seems to be an emotional storytelling, which appears appropriate in drawing out compassion—how can we not help this person?

Advocacy Within the MDT: Use of Re-enactment and Direct Reported Speech to Punctuate Life Stories

Gatekeeping also occurs regarding the services the team offer to service users already well established in their team. This is shown in Extract 2 where they are discussing a service user whose mother is concerned that her child is not being sufficiently challenged at his current school and as such one member of the team (present in the meeting but does not speak in this extract) is going to arrange activities for him over the school holidays, which have already started. This discussion prompts the initiation of a story that uses direct reported speech and re-enactment to argue for additional support for the service user and their family.

Extract 2 Gatekeeping of Resources Within a Service

```
1    DAV:    and Amelia's made a referral to our team because they

2            were sort=of

3            (.) hi↑gher risks than his then I suppose his activity

4            leve↓ls (.) and Rainbow house just focus purely nine to

5            five Monday to Friday

6    SHE: but like the school holidays start now,

7    HOL: they've star[ted]

8    SHE:                [you]know actu:↑ally we could be not being

9         able to see this situation for a

10   DAV: hmm mm

11   SHE: few weeks (.) by which point by the time anything has

12        happe↓ne:d=

13   DAV: mmm

14   SHE: =the school holidays are over=

15   DAV: no of course yeah

16   SHE: =and this man been £that's one thing that's very

17        predictable=

18   DAV: mmm

19   SHE: =is the school holidays£

20   DAV: mmm

21   LIZ: and Danielle Jones she's usually pretty good at
```

```
22        arr:an↓ging ex:tra support if the family's not getting
23        extra support at home
24   DAV: she's not
25   JAN: Danielle had
26   SHI: [>°she did try to organise respite°<]
27   JAN: [ye:ah ye:ah Danielle] had organised a personal budget
28   DAV: yeah
29   JAN: and thought that mum was managing the personal budget
30        but then actually when Amelia and Anne have taken o:ver
31        what they've found is mum has the budget but she doesn't
32        know how to u:se it (.)
33   DAV: mmm
34   JAN: so I think it's kind of >they've said to mum here's your
35        budget off you g:o< and then mums kinda like I don't know
36        what I'm buying with i:t↑
37   SHE: yeah yeah
38   JAN: so I think there's been a bit of a break down
```

This example of advocacy is again produced through the telling of a story, though this time is produced more collaboratively. Dav introduces the referral in lines 1–5. In line 6, She produces a contrastive 'but' which seems to indicate trouble with the upcoming statement 'te school holidays start now'. Again, on line four, six, seven, nine and eleven, She states that the referral for the school holidays has come too late for the team to be able to provide an effective service. On lines 13 and 15, She jokes that one thing that can be relied on is the school holidays. Mockery like this has been linked to disaffiliation (Haugh, 2010). It seems as if 'school holidays' are constructed as having negative connotations for the service user and the family. The case for the school holidays as a problem is rejected at line 21 when Liz interjects suggesting that Danielle is 'pretty good at arranging extra support' suggesting the service user's needs have already been met by services elsewhere, gatekeeping the allocation of further resources. However Jan then joins in at line 26 'Danielle had yeah yeah Danielle had organised a personal budget' in overlap with 'she did try' produced by She, but both of these statements suggest that there is still a problem. Jan goes on to initiate a storied account for why support is still needed. In line 29, she places the action in the past tense—'Danielle thought that mum was managing'. This is contrasted again 'but actually' (line 30). Jan tells the story of how a budget was arranged for the service user's mum, but that when other healthcare professionals followed up they found that the service user's mother was unsure of how to use the budget and summarises this (on line 32) as leading to a breakdown. Again we see reported direct speech in line 34 'they've said to mum here's your budget off you go', and then enactment in lines 35—'mums kinda like I don't know what I'm buying with it'. This seems to enable greater confidence in the upshot assessment of Jan in line 38: 'so I think there's been a bit of a break down'. These stories, then, seem to enable presentation of service users and their families through 'enactments' and emotional illustrations to challenge assumptions made within the team. This story accounts for the extra help the service user and the family needs in an attempt to obtain this from the gatekeepers (in this scenario, She and Liz), and in this way the healthcare professional can be seen to advocate for the service user, pushing for their needs to be met.

Use of Contrast Structures in Advocacy Stories: Reported Experiences of Paid Carers vs the Service User

In our next group of extracts, we examine how stories can be constructed about claims of the best interests of the service user by contrasting the service user's position with that of others (e.g. care staff).

This is illustrated in Extract 3. In this extract, there is a discussion of a new referral to manage the challenging behaviour of a service user. The staff then engage in an elaborative story, which appears to develop a more balanced view of the service user in terms of the reason why the difficulties might have occurred.

Extract 3: Use of Contrast Structures in Advocacy

```
1   JAN:  and then he's go↓ne and it he's had a bad experience but

2         he is continuing to go one day a we:e↓k (.)but the

3         referral tally web was to look at his challenging

4         beh↑aviour=

5   CHI:  [yeah]

6   JAN:  [=but] the causes of his challenging behaviour are

7         <really cle:ar>

8   CHI:  [seems]

9   JAN:  [so ] there's going to be a meeting on the [twenty=]

10  SHE:                                             [wha↑t] are

11        they? what they called?

12  JAN:  =nin↓th (.)[ he was in]

13  CHI:            [communica]

14  JAN:  an environment where he hadn't been introduced

15        [to the staff erm↑]

16  DAV:  [that's right]

17  CHI:  it wasn't graded at all graded at all

18  DAV:  he just went

19  JAN:  yeah £he just went£ [he just turned up=]

20  SHE:                      [he didn't know he was going ]
```

```
21   JAN: =he didn't want to get out of the bus they didn't know

22        how to communicate with [him erm ]

23   SHE:                         [he wasn't] even told he was

24        going was he?

25   JAN: ye:ah there is a lot of probleⱼms

26   CHI: mm

27   JAN: so there is a meeting on the twenty nintⱼh=

28   CHI: [okay]

29   JAN: [=that] Alice and me are going to go to with Sunnydays

30        and mum and

31        [<social care> to look at a longer term plan]

32   SHE: [but we are picking up on po:or ]<social planning>

33        that's esse:ntiaⱼlly
```

In Extract 3, the background is introduced collaboratively. The rationale for referral is completed in lines 3–4. However, this is then discussed by the team which seems to suggest that they already know what is going on—in lines 6–7 Jan states that 'the causes of his challenging behaviour are really clear'. The story telling appears to begin in line 12 with Jan—'he was in an environment...' The story is told collaboratively between Jan, Dav, She and Chi across lines 10 through to 24. The collaborative telling seems to enable little resistance. The three tellers add different assessments each of which increases the 'drama' of the story. It begins with the statement that he 'hadn't been introduced to the environment', supported by Dav. This is upgraded by Chi—'it wasn't graded'—a graded transfer being a planned move from one area to the other. Dav adds 'he just went', and then this is continued by Jan. Jan states 'yeah' affiliating with the trajectory—he 'just went ha just turned up he didn't want to get out of the bus'. This projects the thought of the service user and is contrasted with a projection of the thoughts of the carers—'they didn't know how to communicate with him' (line 22). Jan then presents an upshot on line 25—'yeah there is a lot of problems'. The use of the collaborative support for the very difficult circumstances of the service user, and the upgrade, once again seems to enable a clear identification that there is a concern here for the service, that they then go on to take up. Following the troubles telling (Jefferson....) the upshot is presented in line 27, that there is a meeting, and then there is a collaborative display that the will be 'picking up on poor social planning'.

Key practices here then seem to be the collaborative nature of the storytelling/troubles telling, and the presentation of the service user and the paid carer voices as disparate.

Use of Contrasting Voices in Advocacy Stories: Reported Experiences of the Service User's Family Members vs the Service User

In some cases, advocacy for the service user seemed to be an outcome of the competition between what is in the service user or a family member's interests. In these cases, storytelling was again done in a collaborative fashion between multiple team members. As in the questioning of the paid carer voices in Extract 3, family voices of what is 'OK' for their family member were brought into question through the repetition of voiced actions of the family member. This is illustrated in Extract 4, where a service user went to live with her sister. Her sister's actions are then questioned, and both are described as 'not coping'.

Extract 4: Family Voices

```
1   MAR: she was on quite a lot of medication but I think at

2        some point

3        went to live with family and they [stopped all her=]

4   KAT:                                    [they stopped it ]
```

```
 5   MAR:  =medic↓ation she's living i:n <what isn't an ideal

 6         situation>

 7         she's living in a caravan on a farm with her sis:ter

 8         (3.0)

 9   MAR:  u:m

10         (2.0)

11   MAR:  and I think her sisters certainly got one ch↑il↓d

12   (2.0)

13   KAT:  °>she has<° she's got children with autism

14   MAR:  right

15   KAT   as well

16   MAR:  okay

17   KAT:  mmmm

18   MAR:  so there is a quite a complicated [history of erm

19         (.)abuse]

20   KAT:                              [>yes she's got<]um

21         ye:s she's got she's got bipolar as well a:nd

22         Katherine says she's really

23         difficult to manage (.) >and actually she was in a

24         really settled placement in Tamerton< and then the

25         sister felt that it was more appropriate for her to live

26         at home

27   MAR:  Mmhmm

28   KAT:  So she receives support from > oakhill trust< who

29         aren't coping

30   MAR:  no
```

```
31   KAT:   and it seems like the sister isn't either (.) s:o

32          Katherine has said she's happy to see her again, (0.2)

33          but would like possibly Jamie's support because

34          there's a lot of psychological (2.0)

35          issues there
```

Extract 4 begins immediately after the service user has been introduced to the team. In this extract, the storytelling is used to develop an account that it is appropriate for services to intervene, despite what the family's wishes might have been. Mar begins with an ambiguous description in line 1 that 'she was on a lot of medication at some point', which he contrasts by stating that the family stopped. This is substantiated by Kat in overlap in line 4, which upgrades the telling of this information to the team. Mar continues to describe the living situation as poor. He appears to be reading as there are substantial pauses in the transcript. His telling is again vague in line 11, but supported by Kat in line 13. Mar continues in line 18, summarising the history, and this time Kat in line 20 comes in overlap with an extended turn, giving more background in the form of a diagnostic description ('she's got bipolar') and then an indirect reported speech 'Katherine says she's really difficult to manage' (line 22). Again this use of reported speech as Holt (2017) suggests becomes the prelude to the main issue in the story—that there was a settled placement and then her sister moved her—lines 23–26. A contrast structure is used again in this account—'actually she was in a really settled placement in Tamerton and then her sister felt it was more appropriate for her to live at home'. Although the home situation is not directly critiqued, the contrast structure makes it out to be difficult from the prior more settled situation. These contrasts seem to enable the upshot to be presented without being challenged—'she receives support from Oakhill trust who aren't coping, and it seems like the sister isn't either'.

This extract is organised in a similar way to the prior storytellings, with a background, and build to a significant event or trouble that is punctuated with reported feelings in this case. However, this storytelling is more delicately produced. It appears that no clinician in the room has directly spoken to the sister, and her situation is delicately inferred through discussion of action, or with the qualification 'seems'.

Summary

Advocacy occurs throughout MDT meetings, as each clinician presents and discusses the needs of service users. However, there were particular moments in meetings where barriers to meeting the service user's needs were identified. In these instances, clinicians tended to engage in storytelling—they offered some background and historical events that supported the teller's claim to what the service user needed. These tellings could be to advocate for the service user:

1. where service resources might be limited—for example to engage with a service user who could also be offered services from Adult Mental Health services (which were separate to Learning Disability Services);
2. to advocate for additional support; or
3. to advocate for a service user where either paid carers or family members were considered as being unsupportive to the service user's needs.

These tellings also drew on specific conversational devices in order to enhance the persuasive nature of these tellings. These included:

1. the use of the clinician's personal emotions 'it makes me sad';
2. indirect reported speech;
3. direct reported speech; and
4. contrast structures.

These features were used to 'punctuate' the main tenets of the argument embedded in the storytelling. These stories seemed to embellish the personal meaning, rather than just a diagnostic-based meaning for the service user. Diagnosis was used, as in Extract 4, but here it seemed more as a contrast between the clinician's knowledge and the family's 'feeling' of what was best for the service user. In these tellings, then, epistemics did feature—but the epistemic stance of the MDT or any individual team members were not on its own sufficient to exert power in these cases to immediately propose a course of action without the prior storyteller providing a persuasive account. This building of an account might exemplify the rationale presented by NHS England (2014) for using MDTs—that a more 'holistic' understanding of service users can be developed. Certainly, these storytellings made to the team, and the consequent challenges received, seemed to make the storyteller accountable for the opinion that they offered. Or, if we reverse this, they could be considered to be displaying their accountability through the telling of the story.

A further feature arising from the discussion of advocacy in this chapter was the way in which this was conducted individually or conjointly. In the initial two examples presented here, advocacy stories were presented by one main individual. In these examples, the conversation project appeared to be to persuade the team of the outcome, and a greater number of emotional plea's were witnessed. In the later extracts, where advocacy was around those outside of the team preventing the service users' needs being addressed, there were a greater number of conjoint tellings. It is arguable that these conjoint tellings were more difficult to refute, and teams might reflect on how to ensure that all voices are heard in these debates over external concerns.

Recommendations for Interprofessional Working

- To advocate for a service user, the use of reported speech and personal emotion can be helpful within a Community Learning Disability Setting. Direct reported speech from the service user is difficult to refute as it is as if the service user's opinion is directly brought into the room. Personal emotion may signify compassion, in a healthcare system claiming to be compassionate.

- Conjointly told stories can have greater impact in advocating for service users.
- Where conjoint stories are told, it might be advisable to leave space for others also to comment.

References

Booth, T., & Booth, W. (1996). Sounds of silence: Narrative research with inarticulate subjects. *Disability and Society, 11*(1), 55–69.

Campagna, K. D. (2013). Who will be the patient advocate on a multidisciplinary team? *Hospital Pharmacy, 48*(2), 90–92. http://doi.org/10.1310/hpj4802-90.

Gluyas, H. (2015). Patient-centred care: Improving healthcare outcomes. *Nursing Standard, 30*(4), 50–57.

Griffiths, L., & Hughes, D. (1994). "Innocent parties" and "disheartening" experiences: Natural rhetoric's in neuro-rehabilitation admissions conferences. *Qualitative Health Research, 4*(4), 385–410.

Hansson, E., Ekman, I., Swedberg, K., Wolf, A., Dudas, K., Ehlers, L., & Olsson, L. (2015). Person-centred care for patients with chronic heart failure—A cost-utility analysis. *European Journal of Cardiovascular Nursing*. https://doi.org/10.1177/1474515114567035.

Haugh, M. (2010). Jocular mockery, (dis)affiliation, and face. *Journal of Pragmatics, 42*, 2106–2119.

Henry, L., & Gudjonsson, G. (1999). Eye-witness memory and suggestibility in children with mental retardation. *American Journal of Mental Retardation, 104*(6), 491–508.

Hepburn, A., & Potter, J. (2007). Crying receipts: Time, empathy, and institutional practice. *Research on Language and Social Interaction, 40*(1), 89–116. https://doi.org/10.1080/08351810701331299.

Holt, E. (2017). Indirect reported speech in storytelling: Its position. *Design, and Uses, Research on Language and Social Interaction, 50*(2), 171–187. https://doi.org/10.1080/08351813.2017.1301302.

Jefferson, G. (1984). Transcript notation. In J. M. Atkinson & J. Heritage (Eds.), *Structures of social action: Studies in conversation analysis* (pp. ix–xvi). Cambridge: Cambridge University Press.

Mandelbaum, J. (2013). Storytelling in conversation. In J. Sidnell & T. Stivers (Eds.), *Handbook of conversation analysis* (pp. 492–508). Cambridge: Cambridge University Press.

McGrath, P., Holewa, H., & McGrath, Z. (2006). Nursing advocacy in an Australian multidisciplinary context: Findings on medico-centrism. *Scandinavian Journal of Caring Science, 20*(4), 394–402.

Pilnick, A., Clegg, J., Murphy, E., & Almack, K. (2010). Questioning the answer: Questioning style, choice and self-determination in interactions with young people with intellectual disabilities. *Sociology of Health and Illness, 32*(3), 415–436.

Sklar, M., Aarons, G., O'Connell, M., Davidson, L., & Groessl, E. (2015). Mental health recovery in the patient-centered medical home. *American Journal of Public Health, 105*(9), 1926–1934.

Stone, S. (2008). A retrospective evaluation of the impact of the Planetree patient-centered model of care on inpatient quality outcomes. *Health Environments Research and Design Journal, 1*(4), 55–69.

12

Concern Constructions in Multidisciplinary Team Meetings: Risk or Patient Focused?

Madeleine Tremblett

Introduction

Collaborative working is recognised as important throughout world-wide healthcare systems (Mickan, Hoffman, & Nasmith, 2010). Although there has been a lack of clarity on what the definition of collaboration is in a healthcare context, the concept is cited as important for interprofessional working to deliver benefits to patients (Zwarenstein, Goldman, & Reeves, 2009). A common implementation of interprofessional working in the UK has been the organisation of professionals into multidisciplinary teams (MDT). Despite the implementation of these teams, how collaboration is actually achieved between professionals is less understood. Discursive methods are one potential way to understand what collaboration may look like and how it is performed by healthcare professionals (see Chapter 2).

Much research on collaboration in healthcare teams has focused on what the barriers and facilitators are to achieving collaborative working.

M. Tremblett (✉)
School of Psychology, University of Plymouth, Plymouth, UK
e-mail: madeleine.tremblett@plymouth.ac.uk

© The Author(s) 2018
C. Smart and T. Auburn (eds.), *Interprofessional Care and Mental Health*,
The Language of Mental Health, https://doi.org/10.1007/978-3-319-98228-1_12

Predominantly, conclusions have been drawn from semi-structured interviews with team members. For example, Supper, Catala, Lustmaan, Chemla, Bourgueil, (2014) review of previous studies on interprofessional collaboration in primary care teams highlighted that regular structured meetings facilitate collaboration. Key barriers identified were safeguarding of role responsibilities and differences in approach to treatment. These barriers are of interest when considering that the point of a MDT is to bring together different perspectives on treatment options to determine the best course of action. In other words, the conflicting ideas that team members may bring are meant to lead to a discussion of all potential options so that the best treatment option for the patient is reached. Thus, it is important to consider how these professionals bring these differences of opinion to each other and if it is really a potential barrier to them collaborating or part of the collaborating process. However, considering these conclusions have been drawn from retrospective interviews about meetings, what may feel conflictual could be less so in the moment. Instead, they may actually lead to holistic and collaborative decisions being reached (Belanger & Rodriguez, 2008). Yet, very few studies have examined the process of collaboration when it is meant to occur—in meetings between healthcare professionals. Belanger and Rodriguez (2008) suggest that examining collaboration as it occurs may provide a better insight into the process.

An understanding of the collaborative working process in intellectual (learning) disability (I(L)D) services is equally missing, but perhaps is even more necessary than other healthcare areas. Services provided to adults with I(L)D in the UK have frequently come under scrutiny for poor practice and cases of abuse (cf. Mencap, 2007; services in Cornwall, Commission for Healthcare Audit and Inspection, 2006; Winterbourne View hospital, DoH, 2012). These reports all highlight that there is often an absence of effective multidisciplinary working, which is recurrently emphasised to achieve safe and personalised support for service users (DoH, 2012, 2015a, 2015b). Many of these reviews of services and policy documents highlight communication and working practices between staff as problematic and one factor in major service failures. As such, if an understanding of collaboration in I(L)D services can be provided to staff and policy makers, it could help prevent these problems of risk to service users in the future.

This chapter aims to provide an overview of how discursive methods can be applied to understand collaboration in I(L)D services.

Discourse and Collaboration

My approach to understanding how collaboration is achieved in I(L)D services is based on studying actual multidisciplinary team meetings in a community NHS I(L)D service. Discursive methods, specifically ones based on conversation analysis and its extension discursive psychology, allow a close examination of practices used by participants in conversation. Discursive psychology focuses on the actions performed in talk, with the underlying assumption that the turns in talk, along with non-verbal markers, create and sustain social contexts (see Chapter 2, 4). Although there has been a range of research on interactions between healthcare practitioners and patients (cf. Landmark, Gulbrandsen, & Svennevig, 2015; Maynard & Heritage, 2005; Ten Have, 1991), this method has rarely been used to examine interactions between groups of practitioners before. However, as the MDT team meeting is a predominant site of regular interactions that are intended to be collaborative, this approach can lead to conclusions about collaboration based on actual interactions rather than retrospective accounts of interactions. In this chapter, I will discuss the main outcomes of using this approach. I have focused on examining how staff members obtained collaborative input from other healthcare professionals in the team during the opening sequence of discussing a patient. Specifically, I have examined how the term 'concern' is used in these sequences: (1) that it gains space for collaborative input from team members on a problematic, risk-related patient issue and (2) it also defers the risk for a decision to be an individual's responsibility to a team responsibility. I go on to argue that both these outcomes demonstrate collaboration in situ. However, before discussing the outcomes of the research I will review some relevant background literature.

Opening an issue that needs to be discussed as a 'concern' has previously been identified as having a particular function in an interaction. In a child protection helpline setting, Potter and Hepburn (2003) identified that people wishing to report a potential abuse case would often construct an issue as 'a concern' they had. Potter and Hepburn (2003) argued 'concern' constructions have a specific institutional function for both the caller and the helpline worker, often a child protection officer (CPO). 'Concern' openings notified the recipient (i.e. the CPO) of the beginning of an extended telling sequence, rather than being a self-contained action. Therefore, it provided space in the interaction for the caller to detail the full story and head off an early assessment from the CPO. The 'concern' would then be collaboratively unpacked between the caller and the CPO—becoming a more concrete issue, through elaborative questioning in the interaction. Concern constructions also acknowledge the epistemological differences between the caller and the CPO. They are neutral formations of an issue that demonstrate the caller has not come to a definitive conclusion about the issue yet. As the 'concern' construction allows for discussion, the CPO can bring their knowledge of what should and shouldn't be treated as abuse to help the caller and CPO reach some form of conclusion. In comparison, if a caller refers to the reason they are calling as a 'problem', the reason is treated as something more concrete rather than something to be worked out together between the caller and the CPO. Potter and Hepburn (2003) raised other functions for concern constructions, but these two findings are of most relevance to the use of concern in MDT meetings.

There are some fundamental similarities and differences in Potter and Hepburn's (2003) corpus and the MDT meeting interactions that I have examined. They are both areas in which it is appropriate and expected that the interaction will focus on some issue to do with a person. In the child protection helpline, the differences in epistemic stance are clearly demarcated. The CPO will have epistemic access to what is or isn't a potential child protection issue, but the caller has (normatively) first-hand knowledge of the actual circumstance between the child and the potential abuser. Hence, between the caller and CPO, it is necessary to collaboratively unpack the issue to bring together these different epistemic domains to determine what the right course of action for the child is. In the MDT, the epistemic domains between team members are likely to overlap. The person raising a concern may have access to personal first-hand information about the service user. However, other team members may also have personal knowledge of the service user that can be bought to the discussion. In addition, each team member will have different knowledge that can be bought to the discussion (Heritage, 2012a). For example, a psychiatrist may have an understanding of how medication could be affecting an unusual incontinence problem, whereas a psychologist may have an understanding of anxiety issues that could be affecting the same problem. Anspach (1993) highlighted different knowledge domains in neonatal team decisions, with nurses focusing on their knowledge relating to normative social behaviour, whereas doctors would focus on knowledge relating to scientific information. In comparison with the child protection helpline, the different epistemic domains MDT members bring to the same issue may result in a difference in function of using a 'concern' construction. Yet, they may still demonstrate a way that professionals can gain collaborative input on an issue.

Method

Four hours of previously recorded adult I(L)D MDT meetings were analysed. These specific meetings were 'allocation' meetings, where the team make a decision on whether to allocate their service to service users who have been recently referred by, for example, team members, GPs and social services. To analyse these meetings, conversation analysis (CA) was used. CA is often used in discursive psychology as it examines the action of talk which may demonstrate how psychological concepts are managed by participants in their discourse (Edwards, 1997). CA allows everyday interactional practices to be uncovered through examining the detail of conversation (e.g. intonation, stress, pauses) and what actions the practice has by following the turn-by-turn display of the participant's understanding (Sidnell, 2010).

Following the CA method, first the allocation meetings were orthographically transcribed. All instances of the use of the word 'concern/s' in these meetings were collected ($n = 15$) and Jeffersonian transcription (Jefferson, 1984) was applied these extracts. This level of transcription captures a significant amount of the detail in the talk, including pauses, overlaps and pitch changes. The different patterns of interaction found when using the word concern were subsequently split into different collections of interactions which were performing similar actions (Sidnell, 2010).

Findings

Five different collections of concern constructions were found in the data. These can be split into two main types: constructions that open up discussion to gain input from other team members if a concern is really an issue of risk, and those that do not gain this input (termed non-openers). First, I will review the openers, as these have the function of gaining collaborative input from team members to help determine if a concern is a risk issue.

Openers

Concern constructions that are 'openers' are so because they tend to begin collaborative interaction between team members. Two main types of openers were found in the corpus: speaker-owned concerns and third-party concerns.

Speaker-Owned Concerns

Speaker-owned concerns tend to follow a particular interactional sequence that can be simplified as follows.

Stage One. The preface: At this stage, the team member supplies some background and states 'my concern is..' or similar.
Stage Two. An extended uninterrupted telling: At this stage, the team member will explain the issue in detail to the team.
Stage Three. Interrogative question A: At this stage, the first team member to respond will do so with an interrogative question.
Stage Four. Interrogative question B: At this stage, the next team member (so third speaker) will also respond with an interrogative question.

These stages will be explained through analysis of extract one.

Extract 1: Speaker-Owned Concerns

Cha: Chair; Sky: Skye; Alf: Alfred; Joa: Joan

```
1   Cha:  Luke Chatford? Skye

2   Sky:  er:: yeah so: Luke (.) >has been discharged from hospital

3         now he's back living at ho:me< with Findway care 24-7

4         although (.) um (.) Findway aren't going to be his

5         provider for much longe:r and the reason behind it is

6         because when social care went through their tender

7         process, Findway didn't apply to be part of it °(thing to

8         get a thing for social care to cover this)° and they're

9         also quite expensive, apparently? and so er: the social

10        worker and the solicitor °who was Luke's appointee for-°

11        (.) um looked to see if Luke could you know substitute

12        the costs but he can't it would work out too ↑expensive

13        so that's why their looking for a new provider: ↓um my

14        concerns were that <mum is due to be> discharged from

15        hospital and come home and they were ↑originally sharing

16        a bedroom ↓apparently there are plans to: um move mum

17        into lounge with the hospital bed and the hoist (and all

18        the things) she needs for her needs so >Paul will stay in

19        the bedroom< mum will have the lounge as her bedroom so

20        they have (.) privacy at ni:ght and <mums needs also>

21        needs care from a provider which mums going to pay for

22        herself so mum's still in hospital until a provider can

23        be found which which (   ) um so it's just a real

24        concerning situation, the I've done nursing need

25        assessment and the carer reports that °you know° Luke

26        does s:o much better when mum's not ther:e when mum's not
```

```
27        there? when mum's not interfering with the- the care side
28        of things they know Luke can do that Luke can do this
29        °but° like when they try and go out >mum was saying<
30        don't- don't leave me Luke wants to stay here with me and
31        ↑Luke will respond to that ↓erm so (.) I- I know they
32        have a right to family life and there's no reason why she
33        shouldn't come home but it's just- when she comes home
34        the impact that's going to have ↓I mean it's a tiny house
35        (.) anyway and
36  Alf:  can you evidence that.
37  Sky:  sorry?
38  Alf:  can- can anyone evidence (.) that Luke can function (.)
39        better in isolation than in the company of mum,
40  Sky:  we:ll
41  Alf:  is there enough evidence to
42  Sky:  well Findway aren't very good at doing recording that's
43        the only thing,
44  Alf:  and [then the]re's no point actually
45  Joa:      [but  is:]
46  Joa:  is she going to be significantly cha:nged >↓when she
47        comes ho:me< I mean will it still [b    ]e an issue?
48  Sky:                                    [yeah]
49  Sky:  she's going to fluctuating capacity
```

The first stage of this sequence, the preface (lines 1–13), seems to have a specific interactional role of opening up space in the meeting for the team member to go into detail about the service user issue, without being interrupted. In Extract 1, at line 1 the Chair allocates the floor to Sky to discuss a specific service user (Luke). Sky then begins by providing the details of the events that preface the problems, providing the information that makes the concern relevant in the interaction. This may be similar to the work by Sikveland and Stokoe (2016) in a mediation helpline setting, which found that if the relevance of the mediation had not been established prior to the call taker suggesting a mediation path, people did not engage with suggestions of mediation. Thus, by providing these details prior to stating it is a concern, the speaker is explaining why the concern is relevant.

Sky introduces the problem at line 14 by stating 'my concerns were that'. This statement seems to have a similar action as in storytelling prefaces. Storytelling prefaces in ordinary talk have the action of suspending turn transition until the telling is complete (Stivers, 2013). They work in two ways: (i) they give the recipients a clue as to when the storytelling will be complete and (ii) they convey what stance the teller has on this story and thus what stance the recipient should also take (Stivers, 2013). The preface of 'my concerns were' does both these actions; it shows the recipient that they should find these issues problematic and also shows that the telling is complete once all the issues have been discussed.

Stage two of this sequence, the extended telling (lines 15–37), demonstrates the interactional impact of the preface. There are points in this stage of the extract that it would be appropriate for other team members to take a turn at talk. For example, at line 24 'which which ( )' is a transition relevant place (TRP) due to a trailing off of talk and reduced tempo (Clayman, 2013) and line 32 '↑Luke will respond to that' where the pitch peak on 'Luke' projects an end of a turn construction unit, and thus a TRP (Clayman, 2013). However, there is no transition to another speaker until line 37. I would argue that a transition does not happen earlier than this, as it is only by line 33 the action of the preface is complete; it is clear at this point to recipients that Sky has finished discussing the issues as she repeats a problem already highlighted (first in lines 27 + 28, then in lines 32–33). The trailing off of talk and reduced tempo that occurs in this extended telling also allows for collaboration. It demonstrates a vague unworked course of action and a need for assistance with this issue of potential risk to Luke's independence through the impact of his mum's behaviour.

Stage three of a speaker-owned concern (line 47) moves the turn to another speaker, who tends to ask an interrogative question. An interrogative question at the next turn of talk departs from the storytelling sequence in ordinary conversation. Post-storytelling turns tend to display an evaluative stance towards the story (preferably the one exhibited by the storyteller, Stivers, 2013). However, in the current extract, the post-storytelling turn does not explicitly take the preferred stance; instead, it withholds affiliation with the narrative's stance and interrogates the issue (line 33 'can you evidence that'). Equally, unlike 'ordinary' storytelling sequences, this potentially dispreferred response does not display the normal discourse markers that occur when making a dispreferred response (e.g. delays, prefaces, mitigations and accounts, Pomerantz & Heritage, 2013). Instead, Alf's interrogative shows no delay and is very directive.

In the final stage of a speaker-owned concern, a third speaker will also take a turn with an interrogative question (Joan at line 44 and 45) '… I mean will it still be an issue'. This stage still does not conform to the normal storytelling sequence, as it does not display an evaluative stance. But again, this is not treated as abnormal by Sky in lines 46 and 47, who immediately responds, at one point in overlap ('yeah' at line 46).

In summary, a speaker-owned concern sequence seems to have a number of particular functions in an MDT meeting. The preface seems to give the speaker 'space' in the interaction to lay out the issue to the team, in a similar manner to prefaces in storytelling (Stivers, 2013). However, unlike 'ordinary' conversation, storytelling using a speaker-owned concern preface (e.g. 'my concern') in MDT meetings does not require an uptake of evaluative stance by recipients, instead it has the action of prompting recipient engagement with an issue (i.e. by asking interrogative questions).

Although speaker-owned concerns have an interactional action of opening collaborative discussion when used early in a speaker's telling, if a speaker-owned concern construction is used later in an interaction by a speaker, there is a different action performed. A team member may begin their turn by discussing a service user more generally, explaining why they have been referred to the team. After this general explanation, the team member may go on to state that they are concerned and what reason there is for the concern. Unlike speaker-owned concern constructions that occur at the beginning of a service user discussion, constructions that occur at the end of a discussion can lead to a much earlier transfer of speaker (see line 6 in Extract 2).

Extract 2: Late Speaker-Owned Concern

```
1    Mol:     [↑I'm a bit concerned >as well looking at the

2             patient< profi:le (on)nearly most of the

3             geepee:s assessments are home vis↑ts (.) they

4             ↑don't >seem to be< taking Tom to er appointments

5             very much so=

6    Jim:     =that geepee does go out there a lot

7    Mol:     b↑ut I'm I'm you know↓ they're- they're ↑in ↑the

8             ↑middle ↑of ↓no:↑whe:re it's it's (pfft)>they

9             need to get out< really

10   Kay:     (°bet you loved it didn't ↑you°)
```

The early transfer of speaker suggests it is not interpreted by the recipient as the beginning of a storytelling sequence. Furthermore, there is a tendency for the next turn to be the recipient's evaluative stance, which is often disaffiliative. For example, in line 6, Extract 2, Jim starts to bring trouble to Mol's description of the situation that the home may not be providing appropriate care to their service users. Jim suggests that home visitations are normative behaviour for the GP in question and perhaps not something to be queried. Jim's turn acts to close down this line of reasoning by Mol at an early opportunity. This leads to Mol upgrading the concern to a wider issue about the home not taking service users out in general (line 7). Within this upgrade, Mol completes a self-repair, 'it's it's (pfft) > they need to get out < really' (line 8). This self-repair substitutes a new phrase for the one that was going to be spoken with a stock phrase, closing the discussion. Repairing the talk with a stock phrase seems to demonstrate the speaker's alignment with the non-takeup of the concern by the other members of the team. Thus, a potential boundary condition for speaker-owned constructions opening collaborative discussion is by positioning an assertion that it is a concern at an early opportunity.

Third-Party Concern Constructions

Issues about a service user that are bought to the team on behalf of non-present third party can be presented to the MDT using a concern construction. These tend to have a slightly different trajectory than speaker-owned concerns. Extract 3 is an example of a third-party concern construction found in the data. Dav is presenting a concern previously discussed by Linda who is not present at the meeting. However, unlike speaker-owned concerns, interactants do not allow Dav to complete telling the story of the concern in an uninterrupted way. Instead, two interlocutors also become involved in telling the team about Linda's concerns (Jul at line 6 and Cly at line 10).

Extract 3: Third-Party Concern Construction

```
1    Dav:   Linda I remember in this room we've had °integrated

2           meetings° Li:nda was sat somewhere around the:re and

3           Linda was concerned about this one because she

4           felt >everytime a provider went in< (.) they would

5           s:[abotage it,]

6    Jul:     [sabotage it] yeah

7    Dav:  so it would be like maybe it was all fa- and it was also

8          weird why he was moved back home in the first place he

9          was in an autism provider down at pen-

10   Cly:  and and he was really settled where he was
```

The collaboration with other team members to complete the presentation of the third-party concern may occur due to a higher level of shared knowledge compared to speaker-owned concerns. When a speaker constructs their own concern to the team, recipients cannot be sure that they share knowledge of what the individual's concern is. Thus, it is necessary to allow a speaker to expand on their concern before they can take the appropriate next action. However, some recipients may have been privy to the third-party's concerns from previous interactions. Nonetheless, there is still space allowed in the conversation for collaborative unpacking of the concern until it is hearable that it has been fully presented, so that all recipients in the team gain this knowledge. The space provision afforded by a third-party construction makes them similar to speaker-owned concerns.

The response to a third-party concern construction is not similar to speaker-owned concerns. When the concern is hearably complete, like storytellings, there is an evaluation of the story. This can be seen in Extract 4, which comes 18 lines later in the interaction that began in Extract 3 (in the intervening period, the service users' background and issues with the family are discussed). In Extract 4, the concern construction hearably finishes at line 2, with an upshot of the story by Cly stating 'so they got the money', suggesting there may be a risk that the family are not providing the best care but instead are motivated by potential income. Rather than an immediate affiliative evaluation by a recipient, there is a gap in the interaction at line 3, predicating some trouble in the next turn. The next turn, Rob at line 4, goes on to suggest some other interpretations of the concerns presented. An alternative explanation is sensitively provided by Rob that other circumstances in the service user's background may help explain their parents' behaviour.

Extract 4: Third-Party Concern Construction Continued

```
1   Cly:  -so that (0.5) he could be (David's) paid (.) carer

2         ↓didn't he so °they got the money°

3         (1.6)

4   Rob:  °°I think it's: it's °° (0.3) >as I said (it's sort of)

5         there is this life events< which are going o:n behind

6         the scene
```

Thus, using a third-party concern construction also has a similar impact to using a speaker-owned concern by providing space in a meeting for a risk-related service user problem to be raised; however, there is more of an evaluative stance taken by recipients. The variation in recipient response may be due to the nature of the concern. It is not a personal concern to the speaker, and thus, interrogating them about it is not appropriate. Furthermore, because it is not personal to the speaker, an evaluation may be a more acceptable action. Theoretically, there is no personal face lost by colleagues directly disagreeing with the concern, as the speaker can always refer it back to the third party (as is done later in the interaction by Cly). Equally, the concern is not owned by a member of the present group, so taking an evaluative stance to a non-present member's concern may be more normative as it does not risk disrupting intragroup relationships.

Non-openers

Looking at every instance of the word 'concern' in the corpus found some uses of the term 'concern' that did not lead to a collaborative discussion of a service user concern to determine its legitimacy. However, the use of the term tended to perform an action in the interaction which highlights how it is normatively used as a discussion opener. Below, the three other ways concern was used in the corpus are reviewed.

'No Concern'

When discussing service user issues at times, team members would state that there was 'no concern' (see Extract 5).

Extract 5: Example of a Team Member Using 'No Concern'

```
1    Alf: but there was no concerns about epilepsy at all.

2    Alf: his: carers were reporting issues around forgetfulness,

3         (.)
```

The statement of 'no concern' would often be in relation to one issue that a service user was experiencing. Adults with learning disabilities tend to have complex health needs. Thus, when a professional is describing a service user to the team, a number of these issues are often raised. By stating 'no concern' in relation to a specific issue, as in line 1 in Extract 5, Alf is preventing the recipients from focusing on the issue of epilepsy in their responses. The use of 'no concern' to close a potential focus of the interaction is emphasised in line 1. Alf finishes stating that there are no concerns about the epilepsy with 'at all'. Ending on a negative polarity item (at all) is oriented to a no response (Heritage, Robinson, Elliot, Beckett, & Wilkes, 2007). This section of talk is also marked with a downward final intonation, ending the turn construction unit (TCU). Even though it is an end of a TCU, which is a normative place for a next speaker to begin, there is no change in speaker. It is clear to recipients that though Alf is closing this area as a topic of conversation, he is going on to discuss the main issue to do with the service user. Beginning with mentioning the potential concern (around epilepsy) conforms to the organisational requirement to acknowledge a risk, but offsets the development of a concern construction by revising and tightening the potential problem. This is almost a stepwise entry into the problem, which can be similarly found in advice sequences provided by healthcare visitors (Heritage & Sefi, 1992). Alf's negative declarative of 'no concern at all' takes a knowing epistemic stance, which invites agreement and sequence closure (Heritage, 2012b). Thus, the action of stating that this is 'no concern' highlights that rather than being a concern for the team to discuss, moves the interaction to focus on other issues.

Definitive 'Concern' (i.e. She's/There's a Concern)

In comparison with concern constructions which open up discussion to determine if a concern is a risk issue, the use of 'there's a concern' presents an issue as definitive. Interactions in the team then focus on other issues related to the concern. Extract 6 provides an example of a definitive concern. Initially, the team are discussing if a letter has been sent to query the quality of a handover.

Extract 6: Definitive Concern

```
1   Mark:     Cassandra Bluet↑on

2             (2.0)

3   Sally:    °I think um° that's Josie and Molly did the initial

4             ( ) internal refer↑rals    [(              )]

5   Yvonne:                               [yeah it's it's on]

6                      [bring back=]

7   Mark:     [ye:      ah]

8   Yvonne:   =be↑cause >there's outstanding action of doing of< a

9             writing a letter rega:rding a ha:nd over

10  Josie:    °oh that was: you then was↑n't ↑it°

11  Molly:      yeah >↑I've done it-< °yeah°

12  Mark:     ye↑ah=

13  Molly:    =>↑I've done it ↑aint ↑I<

14  Josie:    yeah (.) I th:ink so:

15  Molly:    ↑ye↑ah to kate to say >there wasn't a good enough<

16            ↑hand↓over it was- it was part of my le:tter that

17            was:=

18  Yvonne:   =right=

19  Molly:    =about we're gunna >do all of these th↑ings< but >by

20            the wa:y< (.) [it  isn't] good enough

21  Yvonne:                 [ah↑o↓kay]                    right

22  Molly:    there's lots of conce:rns here

23  Mark:     yeah

24  Molly:    not lea:st that- [mum's]

25  Mark:                      [mum's] ↑ye↓ah
```

Once there has been clarification of who has done the handover (lines 10–14), there is little explanation about the handover or concern. Although at line 23 Mol mentions a concern, unlike many other concern constructions there is immediate affiliation by a recipient in the interaction (line 24). The use of definitive concern by Mol in line 23 takes a knowing epistemic stance on behalf of the team (Heritage, 2012b), which invites affiliation by the team (seen by Mark in line 24; Lambertz, 2011). A lack of explanation and the immediate affiliation to this point suggest that the 'concerns' have already been discussed by the team. Rather than trying to invite discussion, it acts to formulate and summarise the case as an upshot of what has previously been discussed. As such, the team already have shared knowledge and agreement on the concern. Thus, the use of a definitive concern construction seems to prevent further interaction on whether this is a risk issue for team consideration.

Hypothetical Concern (e.g. If There Was a Concern)

Hypothetical concerns highlight the use of concern constructions as something to open discussion in the team meetings. They are usually used in reference to whether a service user needs to be discussed in later meetings. For an example of this, see Extract 7.

Extract 7: Hypothetical Concern

```
1   Mar:    >do you need to bring that back after you've done the

2           quomid? or will that go into< the dementi:a

3   Dee:    (            )

4   Mar:    okay

5   Dee:    >u- unless there's anything, <concerning

6   Mar:    okay
```

Extract 7 comes at the end of a service user discussion by the team. Mar in line 1 questions whether the service user will need to be 'bought back' to a future meeting after an assessment has been completed (a 'quomid' on line 1). The question is designed to elicit a response that fits with the organisation's (here the I(L)D team) goals. To 'go into the dementia' (line 2) is for the patient to be referred to a different team. The option for this patient to go to another team has been placed as the second option in Mar's question. There is a hierarchy of preference in either/or questions (Antaki & O'Reilly, 2014), with the second option being the preferred option. Positioning the less preferable option first means that interactants have to do more work to state that as their preference. The initial answer by Dee seems to be oriented to the second option (although it is hard to hear on the recording) as she states that she can take it to the team (presumably the dementia team). However, Dee does go on to state at line 5 that bringing it back (the first option) would only be necessary if there was anything 'concerning' as a result of the assessment. This demonstrates how the use of 'concern' can be used to validate choosing the less preferred option. The way a 'hypothetical' concern has been used by Dee also demonstrates a norm in the team that orients to concerns being a valid reason for a group discussion.

The Nature of a Concern in MDT Meetings

The MDT meeting is designed for staff members to discuss issues and problems relating to a service user so it is important to think about what function doing this as a 'concern' may have for team members. In the analysis above, I have discussed how it signals to recipients that there is a 'story' being told by the speaker, and thus, recipients provide the necessary space for the full story to be told before taking a turn. Concern constructions function in a different way to 'storytellings' so that it is not necessary for the recipients to respond with an affiliative assessment of the 'story', i.e. the concern. Instead, with speaker-owned concerns team members often respond with interrogatives to gain more information on the nature of the concern. Alternatively, third-party concern constructions can lead to a dis-affiliative evaluative stance by the recipient. Thus, it is not treated as a story by recipients. Instead, it seems the action of a concern construction is that they provide an opportunity for team members to bring a undecided issue to the MDT (at least for opening concern constructions). The MDT can then work collaboratively to determine if this issue is an actual issue or not, using the range of professional knowledge the team members hold. This function is demonstrated by the recipients' responses to the concern constructions focusing on whether this issue is an actual issue, rather than suggesting potential solutions to the concern (see also Chapter 6 on 'seeking help').

The issues that are presented in concern constructions all relate to potential risk. The risk is to a service user from their current provider or from a family member. For example, in Extract 7, the third-party concern relates to whether family members are only taking care of a service user to gain money, rather than having the service user's best interests at heart. Risk-related issues are particularly sensitive for learning disability services. Historically, major service failures have been linked to risk issues not being properly managed by learning disability services. Thus, potential risks to service users need to be dealt with sensitively by professionals. However, there is an individual cost to raising a potential risk issue (Attree, 2007). There are consequences to a professional if a risk has not been properly assessed but is still raised to safeguarding. Raising something officially as a risk would need to be taken seriously by services, creating a high level of involved work for the service. In the current climate of stretched resources, an unfounded risk referral could be deemed as wasting time for a service. Furthermore, services often need to work in conjunction with providers and family members. If a risk is raised that ends up as unfounded, this may damage the relationship between the service and the perpetrators of potential risk. Finally, at an individual level, a team member's professional judgement may be questioned if it is found that a concern is not actually a risk to a service user. When team members use a concern construction, they can defer the rights of assessment of the risk to the team, rather than being the sole person accountable for the judgement. The deferral of assessment is similar to what was observed by Potter and Hepburn (2003) in their analysis of calls to a child protection helpline. Callers would use concern constructions to defer the right of assessment of the risk to the organisation. Consequently, the use of concern constructions allows the individual professional to be comfortable that they have done something with a 'concern', and that the burden of this 'concern' is no longer held by them as an individual; instead, it is shared with the team.

The ability for team members to share a potential risk to a service user and gain input to assess this risk is one demonstration of how collaboration is achieved between professionals. Collaboration can be seen as teams working together to solve problems and is often conceptualised as such in the literature. This does not happen automatically when team members are bought together, they must perform actions to gain collaborative input from other team members. A concern construction is one way of them being able to get the collaborative input from other members. Furthermore, teams are not there to just share knowledge with one another but also to share the burden of decisions so that the responsibility of the decisions is not purely on the individual. Not only does that move accountability off the individual to the team, but it also ensures that decisions become made through team consensus and thus become more robust decisions. This robustness comes from the different perspectives that the various team members can bring to decision-making. Bringing a range of perspectives to a decision is the main point of a MDT and thus any way that professionals can capitalise on gaining this variety of perspectives, from using a concern construction, for example helps a MDT achieve this aim.

Recommendations for Interprofessional Team Working

Prefacing the presentation of a potential risk issue by stating 'my concern is..' (or similar) can help provide a safe space in a team meeting to fully detail the circumstances underpinning the concerns that are held. Using a speaker-owned concern construction can then lead to other members of the team collaboratively helping determine the plausibility of the concern, drawing on a wide range of knowledge bases.

It is important that these concerns are raised early in the interaction to gain collaborative input. Any additional concerns that get raised later in the interactional sequence may not be afforded the same discussion due to an organisational preference for progressivity to the next case. Thus, if additional circumstances are concerning in the course of a service user discussion, it could be helpful to arrange a list of additional concerns to get logged onto a service user's case file so that they do not get missed.

References

Anspach, R. (1993). *Deciding who lives: Fateful choices in the intensive-care nursery*. Berkeley: University of California Press.

Antaki, C., & O'Reilly, M. (2014). Either/or questions in child psychiatric assessments: The effect of the seriousness and order of the alternatives. *Discourse Studies, 16*(3), 327–345.

Attree, M. (2007). Factors influencing nurses' decisions to raise concerns about care quality. *Journal of Nursing Management, 15*, 392–402.

Belanger, E., & Rodriguez, C. (2008). More than the sum of its parts? A qualitative research synthesis on multidisciplinary primary care teams. *Journal of Interprofessional Care, 22*(6), 587–597.

Clayman, S. E. (2013). Turn-construction units and the transition-relevance place. In J. Sidnell & T. Stivers (Eds.), *The handbook of conversation analysis* (pp. 150–166). Chichester: Blackwell.

Commission for Healthcare Audit and Inspection. (2006). *Joint investigation into the provision of services for people with learning disabilities at Cornwall Partnership NHS Trust*. Retrieved from http://webarchive.nationalarchives.gov.uk/20060502043818/, http:/healthcarecommission.org.uk/_db/_documents/cornwall_investigation_report.pdf.

DoH. (2012). *Transforming care: A national response to Winterbourne View Hospital*. Retrieved from https://www.gov.uk/government/uploads/system/uploads/attachment_data/file/213215/final-report.pdf.

DoH. (2015a). *No voice unheard, no right ignored—A consultation for people with learning disabilities, autism and mental health conditions*. Retrieved from https://www.gov.uk/government/uploads/system/uploads/attachment_data/file/409816/Document.pdf.

DoH. (2015b). *Government response to no voice unheard, no right ignored—A consultation for people with learning disabilities, autism and mental health conditions*. Retrieved from https://www.gov.uk/government/uploads/system/uploads/attachment_data/file/475155/Gvt_Resp_Acc.pdf.

Edwards, D. (1997). *Discourse and cognition*. London: Sage.

Heritage, J. (2012a). Epistemics in action: Action formation and territories of knowledge. *Reseach on Language and Social Interaction, 45*(1), 1–29.

Heritage, J. (2012b). Epistemics in conversation. In J. Sidnell & T. Stivers (Eds.), *The handbook of conversation analysis* (pp. 370–394) Oxford, UK: Wiley-Blackwell.

Heritage, J., Robinson, J. D., Elliot, M. N., Beckett, M., & Wilkes, M. (2007). Reducing patients' unmet concerns in primary care: The different one word can make. *Journal of General Internal Medicine, 22*(10), 1429–1433.

Heritage, J., & Sefi, S. (1992). Dilemmas of advice. Aspects of the delivery and reception of advice in interactions between health visitors and first time mothers. In P. Drew & J. Heritage (Eds.), *Talk at work* (pp. 359–417) Cambridge: Cambridge University Press.

Jefferson, G. (1984). Transcription notation. In J. Atkinson & J. Heritage (Eds.), *Structures of social interaction*. New York: Cambridge University Press.

Lambertz, K. (2011). Back-channelling: The use of *yeah* and *mm* to portray engaged listenership. *Griffith Working Papers in Pragmatics and Intercultural Communication, 4* (1/2), 11–18.

Landmark, A. M. D., Gulbrandsen, P., & Svennevig, J. (2015). Whose decision? Negotiating epistemic and deontic rights in medical treatment decisions. *Journal of Pragmatics, 78*, 54–69.

Maynard, D. W., & Heritage, J. (2005). Conversation analysis, doctor-patient interaction and medical communication. *Medical Education, 39*, 428–435.

Mencap. (2007). *Death by indifference*. Retrieved from https://www.mencap.org.uk/sites/default/files/2016-06/DBIreport.pdf.

Mickan, S., Hoffman, S. J., & Nasmith, L. (2010). Collaborative practice in a global health context: Common themes from developed and developing countries. *Journal of Interprofessional Care, 24*(5), 495–502.

Pomerantz, A., & Heritage, J. (2013). Preference. In J. Sidnell & T. Stivers (Eds.), *The handbook of conversation analysis* (pp. 210–228). Chichester: Blackwell.

Potter, J., & Hepburn, A. (2003). "I'm a bit concerned"—Early actions and psychological constructions in a child protection helpline. *Research on Language and Social Interaction, 36*(3), 197–240.

Sidnell, J. (2010). *Conversation analysis: An introduction*. Chichester: Wiley-Blackwell.

Sikveland, R. O., & Stokoe, E. (2016). Dealing with resistance in initial intake and inquiry calls to mediation: The power of 'willing'. *Conflict Resolution Quarterly, 33*(3), 235–254.

Stivers, T. (2013). Sequence organisation. In J. Sidnell & T. Stivers (Eds.), *The handbook of conversation analysis* (pp. 191–209). Chichester: Blackwell.

Supper, I., Catala, O., Lustmanm, M., Chemla, C., Bourgueil, Y., & Letrilliart, L. (2014). Interprofessional collaboration in primary health care: A review of facilitators and barriers perceived by involved actors. *Journal of Public Health, 37*(4), 716–727.

Ten Have, P. (1991). Talk and institution: A reconsideration of the 'asymmetry' of doctor-patient interaction. In D. Boden & D. H. Zimmerman (Eds.), *Talk and social structure: Studies in ethnomethodology and conversation analysis* (pp. 138–163). Cambridge: Polity Press.

Zwarenstein, M., Goldman, J., & Reeves, S., (2009). Interprofessional collaboration: Effects of practice-based interventions on professional practice and healthcare outcomes. *Cohrane Database Systematic Review, 8*(3), CD000072.

13

Listening to 'Early Intervention in Psychosis Teams' Talk About Psychosis and Its Meaning: The Perspective of Those with Lived Experience of Psychosis

Claire Whiter, Ben Durkin and Ashley Tauchert

Introduction

This chapter explores how people with lived experience of psychosis, respond to interprofessional team discussions on the topic of psychosis. Here, we present summaries of conversations which occurred during the process of analysing transcripts from focus groups held with staff from Early Intervention in Psychosis Teams (EI) as part of Claire's doctoral research project. Speaking from our individual perspectives as people with lived experience of psychosis (Ben and Ashley) and experience as a former member of staff within an EI team (Claire), we share our responses to the transcripts. These responses include our immediate reactions to the content and the discursive tools used by staff, as well as our reflections on service provision, its sociopolitical context and related philosophical considerations. They provide a critical insight into how staff from different

C. Whiter (✉)
Livewell Southwest, Plymouth, UK

B. Durkin · A. Tauchert
Peer Support Organisation, Exeter, UK

© The Author(s) 2018
C. Smart and T. Auburn (eds.), *Interprofessional Care and Mental Health*,
The Language of Mental Health, https://doi.org/10.1007/978-3-319-98228-1_13

professions collectively constitute psychosis. They further allow reflection on how service users and experts by experience can effectively contribute to discursive research and enhance its impact. By presenting subsequent reflections on our involvement in the research, we hope to encapsulate our individual experiences of participation in the project and demonstrate the rich possibilities of this method of involvement.

To begin, in the project overview we describe the context within which focus groups with staff involved in interprofessional working were held, experts by experience were recruited and transcripts initially discussed. We then present summaries of a series of conversations between us in response to the transcripts of the focus group discussions. These conversations were responsive to the discursive repertoires, subject positions and ideological dilemmas (Edley, 2001) identified in the data analysis and which have enabled us to make recommendations for interprofessional working. Finally, we each provide individual reflections on our involvement together and summarise with conclusions and recommendations for collaboration between researchers and people with lived experience of psychosis.

Project Overview

Psychosis and Early Intervention Services

'Psychosis' is a term that is often used to refer to experiences which appear out of touch with reality. For example, hearing and seeing things that other people do not, having extremely suspicious thoughts and holding beliefs which others find strange (Cooke, 2015). Psychosis is also a diagnostic term used by psychiatric services to indicate particular treatment pathways. There has been much debate around what constitutes psychosis, as this may be considered to be highly dependent on the perspective of the diagnostician. Many perceptual and thought disturbances which may be considered 'psychotic' are also experienced by members of the general population whose lives may not be as severely affected as those who access the support of psychiatric services (Kelleher, Jenner, & Cannon, 2010). Research into the health and social outcomes for people experiencing psychosis indicates that the earlier interventions (social, psychological or medical) are provided, the better the likelihood is for recovery (Birchwood, Fowler, & Jackson, 2000). It is on this principle that Early Intervention in Psychosis (EI) Services have been created. These specialist multi-disciplinary mental health teams aim to identify and provide interventions for people experiencing a first episode of psychosis and their families.

Perspectives on the conceptualisation, identification and treatment of psychosis can be passionate and conflicting. Competing discourses around psychosis abound within academic texts (Boyle, 2002; Read, Mosher, & Bentall, 2004) and across social and popular media (e.g. Williams, 2012). As EI services are considered to bridge traditional and recovery-orientated practice (Roberts, 2006), these service settings were considered fertile ground for multiple evolving understandings of psychosis which may range on a spectrum from viewing psychosis as a collection of meaningless symptoms of illness to being a meaningful response to life events (Longden, 2013).

Research Aims

The research aims arose from Claire's experience of encountering a service user's personal narrative of psychosis which presented the experience as personally meaningful; challenging her perception of psychosis as an illness triggered by stress, with apparently meaningless content. Reflecting on her sense of discomfort and in her experience as a staff member within an EI team, she questioned the availability of discourses of meaningfulness within mental health service settings and the opportunities available to explore alternative narratives of psychosis, other than those of illness. Of particular interest to this project, were the trans-disciplinary constructs of psychosis and how these are deployed within an EI multi-disciplinary team setting. A critical discursive psychology (CDP) approach was chosen to explore the discourses around psychosis with the specific aim of examining the idea of the meaningfulness of the experience of psychosis, i.e. how might staff consider psychosis to be personally meaningful to those living with psychosis, and the meanings that an individual might attribute to, within and through their psychotic experiences (Roberts, 2000).

Method

This project strongly endorsed the principle of patient and public involvement in health-based research (NIHR, 2018). During the initial stages of the research, we therefore consulted with those who had both lived experience of psychosis and of accessing statutory mental health services. In addition, Claire felt it was imperative to include the perspective of people with lived experience to enhance the reflexivity of the researchers and to support a better-informed consideration of the research implications. She approached a local collective of people with experiences described as psychosis, to discuss the initial research idea and formulate focus group questions. Two members of the collective (Ben and Ashley) continued to be involved as consultants in the analysis. Involvement of the research consultants evolved as the research progressed, from consultation on the initial research idea to participate in reflective discussions in response to the transcripts.

Six multi-disciplinary EI teams (each team comprising a range of nursing, social work, occupational therapy, psychology and support worker staff) from one NHS trust were approached to participate in the research. A focus group method was chosen to allow the topic of meaningfulness to be introduced by asking staff what comes to their minds with the statement: 'psychosis can be meaningful' and what they do or say to work with meanings of psychosis. A focus group was held for each of the three teams who chose to participate, facilitated by Claire. There were representatives from a range of professions within each group. Group A comprised four Community Psychiatric Nurses (CPNs), one student nurse and one social worker. Group B comprised five CPNs, one Occupational Therapist (OT) student, one social worker, one OT and one support worker. Group C comprised of four CPNs, one OT, one clinical psychologist and one support worker. Although invited, no psychiatrists participated in the focus groups.

Method of Analysis

Orthographic transcriptions from each focus group were analysed by adopting a Critical Discursive Psychology perspective, exploring how staff constructions of psychosis and meaningfulness might be socially, organisationally or politically informed (Edley, 2001; Taylor, 2013). Changing understandings of psychosis, psychological research evidence and current mental health service contexts form the social environment of EI teams. The process of analysing talk highlights discursive resources such as particular words, phrases or ways of talking about a topic. These resources can be used both to position staff and service users and in turn, create dilemmas for staff. By referring to the analytical constructs of linguistic or interpretative repertoires (Potter & Wetherell, 1987), ideological dilemmas (Billig, Condor, Edwards, Gane, Middleton, & Radley, 1988) and subject positions (Wetherell, 1998), we considered the complexity of both the social environment of the EI team and how meanings of psychosis are constructed in interaction within this environment.

Transcripts were read independently by Claire and three research supervisors, and then decisions were made collectively about whether ways of talking about identified topics were repertoires, whether they represented dilemmas or subject positions by referring to how they were used by speakers in the transcripts. During this process, transcripts were also read independently by Ben and Ashley who noted down their responses to and reflections on the transcripts. Ben, Ashley and Claire then met together on three separate occasions to discuss each transcript in turn, reflecting on the content and topics and considering implications for practice. Written notes were made during these discussions and later typed up.

Analytical Constructs: Repertoires, Dilemmas and Subject Positions

'Linguistic repertoires' were first used by Potter and Wetherell (1987) to describe ways of talking about a topic that are used by a particular culture or group of people and might include particular phrases, keywords or metaphors that are repeatedly referred to. They emphasised that repertoires were action oriented in so far as a version of the world is discursively constructed for interpersonal and ideological purposes.

The term 'ideological dilemma' was used by Billig et al. (1988) to describe occasions when two or more commonly held beliefs or ideals within a culture appear to contradict each other. These ideals may be intrinsic and long established and the dilemmatic nature of their contradiction can reveal the complexity of the sociopolitical climate that group members have to negotiate. Billig et al. illustrate this with examples of contradictory common-sense ideologies such as: 'absence makes the heart grow fonder' but 'out of sight is out of mind'.

The analytical concept of 'subject positions' was introduced by Davies and Harré (1990) to describe how language may be used to position people rhetorically or ascribe them a particular identity by referencing certain values. Bell (2010) explores this concept with reference to 'healthy eating', by describing how a person identified as a 'healthy eater', is positioned here rhetorically by values around health. Thus, subject positions can be used to explore the operation of power by considering whose interests this positioning serves and from where value-based judgments may have come.

Each of these three analytic resources are not mutually exclusive, and a linguistic repertoire may also highlight an ideological dilemma or be used to achieve subject positioning. For example, a discursive repertoire around labelling service users as 'psychotic' could also produce ideological dilemmas for staff both wanting to avoid labelling and needing to assign labels in order to provide a service. This might then be used to produce subject positions for different team members, for example 'those that support the use of labels' and 'those that don't'.

Reflective Discussions

Our discussions on the transcripts allowed for consideration of what was left 'unsaid' in the focus groups but might be considered important from the perspective of lived experience. This informed our interpretation of the rhetorical use of language within the transcripts and provided ideas for future research directions. These discussions provided an insightful and important reflective lens from the perspective of lived experience.

Findings

The initial analysis of the focus group interactions identified four main repertoires which captured meaningfulness in relation to psychosis: labelling, life experiences, historical understandings and service priorities. These repertoires each functioned to position service users, staff and sometimes the service itself. Several of the repertoires also produced ideological dilemmas for staff. These repertoires are summarised in Table 13.1.

Extracts from the transcripts are presented later in this chapter to illustrate both the themes of discursive repertoire identified in the full analysis and how these stimulated reflective discussions between the lead researcher and research consultants.

Table 13.1 Four main repertoires

Repertoires	Description of repertoire and how it was used by staff
Labelling	Labelling presented an ideological dilemma for staff who both wanted to de-stigmatise, therefore avoided using the 'label' of psychosis, and needed to use diagnostic terms to provide a service. This dilemma had implications for staff's positioning of themselves and service users, from 'collaborators' to 'us and them'
Psychosis can be a meaningful life experience	Staff described how psychosis may be an impactful life event, may be contextualised by life events or may serve a purpose for someone's life. This allowed staff to position themselves as detectives looking for clues to make sense of these experiences
Historical understandings of psychosis	Staff constructed a repertoire to describe historical ways of working which positioned service users as 'ill' and staff attempting to explore psychotic content as 'colluding'. This was used to distance themselves from historical practices, positioning themselves as 'pioneers'
Service priorities	Repertoires around service priorities were constructed from descriptions of how other parts of the mental health service operate. These were positioned as having limited understandings of meaning due to having limited resources and different priorities

Summaries of Discussions with Research Consultants

Reflective consultation meetings to discuss the transcripts produced further data which have allowed us to make recommendations for inter-professional working. We found that the process of meeting regularly to read the transcripts together produced a rich, lively discussion between us, from which arose ideas for what we each considered psychosis to mean, how we feel EI teams might work and reflections on more traditional service approaches towards psychosis. Although these discussions arose in a freeform and organic way and did not constitute formal analysis of the data, they could be related to the four repertoires that were identified through the formal analysis.

In the next section, we present summaries of these discussions which relate to the repertoires identified, together with extracts from the transcripts. Alongside this, we present our broader discussion stimulated by these repertoires.

Labelling

Related to the theme of labelling, we observed that staff placed emphasis on 'finding a shared language'. We reflected how in our experience as service users, it was helpful to learn the language of psychiatry, in order to 'get a good deal'. We felt that using psychiatric terms can be levelling and constructive. In our view, there are multiple languages for the experience of psychosis, all of them valid, the problem comes when one dominates and attempts to silence all others. We agreed with the focus group staff that it is important to find a shared language and considered metaphors to be a vehicle for shared meaning. However, we felt that metaphors can get imposed from the mental health service and wondered if they can also come from the side of the service user. The experience itself may be a metaphor and expression of a particular way of constituting psychosis; we felt that being able to discuss the experience freely and openly without fear means it can be possible to unpick more fully.

A further aspect of the labelling repertoire was around 'insight'. We felt that staff did not want to do damage with their use of this word.

However, we reflected that from each of our experiences, 'insight' is often used within mental health services to suggest that someone does not understand their own thoughts. We felt it was a shame that the word insight has become a difficult term for staff, as it gets used to mean that 'you don't know you're ill' and that a person who has insight means 'you have accepted that you are ill'. We suggested that insight can sometimes feel like a line you are supposed to cross to reach 'normal'.

Within the labelling repertoire, there was an orientation to avoiding the use of the word 'schizophrenia'. We conceptualised this orientation as an ideological dilemma:

Extract 1: Staff Focus Group A

```
Finn[1]   '…because there's a lot of stigma around in the media
          isn't there and misunderstanding about psychosis and
          schizophrenia, you know that word that we try not to
          use or there's a lot of ignorance about so I guess
          yeah working with people around normalising
          experiences…' (A:226-231)
```

We talked about the implications of this for people experiencing psychosis and/or having received a diagnosis of schizophrenia. We recognised, that for some people, schizophrenia can be viewed with pride; there may be a sense of ownership. We reflected that historically mental health staff have focused on service users accepting this diagnosis, linking it with insight, and now it feels as if they want to take it away. We wondered whether avoiding using the term also makes it unspeakable and therefore further stigmatising. During our discussion, we thought that trying to get people to accept the idea that they are psychotic is not really necessary, instead from our experience, the focus should be on psycho-geography or a 'rudimentary map'. In other words, we thought that the staff appeared focused on identification rather than exploration of psychotic experiences.

Historical Understandings of Psychosis

We observed that staff made frequent reference to the methods and approaches used when working with psychosis, and we discussed how this may also relate to the changes in historical understandings of psychosis. Staff labelled the advice they had received earlier in their mental health careers as being part of the 'old regime' which restricted psychosis to be narrowly understood as meaning 'illness'. Staff repeatedly drew upon 'the old regime' to highlight how approaches in EI are different, by distancing themselves from historical understandings and positioning themselves as 'pioneers'.

Within the transcripts, we noticed that timelines appeared to be an often-cited method for working with psychosis and we wondered whether this might be framing the experience in terms of cause and effect. Our concern was that causation might then be the focus of work, rather than meaning. A timeline, in our view, places a focus on the linear; whereas in our personal experience, psychosis is an explosion of meaning, and it is simultaneous and multi-dimensional. The timeline feels reductionist, though plotting can be helpful if you don't know where to start.

The therapeutic relationship was referenced a number of times by staff throughout the transcripts. There was an interesting aspect of the repertoire around 'them and us' which produced dilemmas and positioning for staff and service users:

Extract 2: Staff Focus Group C

Nicky: 'I think of EI, of the teams I've worked in, the boundaries are not non-existent, because we have to protect ourselves professionally but really, the whole them and us stuff is very...'

Paula: '...but there isn't a them and us to me, there isn't a them and us'

Nicky: 'No'

Paula: 'Well, there is in that they are asking us for help'

(C: 604–611)

We agreed that there has to be 'them and us' in order for the teams to exist, it is an important boundary, and we felt that saying there is no them and us makes the boundary blurred. Our reactions to reading about them and us in the transcript were of feeling both offended and reassured by the honesty of staff. We acknowledged that when you become the 'them', there is no choice; staff have to visit you at home. In our experiences of receiving mental health services, if people receiving the service miss appointments, they may get into trouble, and if staff miss them, there appears to be no problem.

Staff also drew upon the stress-vulnerability model within the transcripts as an explanatory framework for understanding psychosis. We thought that the language of 'vulnerability' might be interpreted as being 'weak' and unable to handle stress. We questioned the notion that anyone might experience psychosis at some point in their lives, by the simple fact that they don't. Again, we felt that this model demonstrated an implicit assumption that 'having psychosis' is something negative and wrong.

Reading staff talk about the support they provide service users in EI settings, led to much reflection of our own experiences of mental health services. From our experience, we have found that staff have traditionally aimed to stop us from having these experiences and exploring them was seen as not relevant, or even colluding or dangerous. Historically, there has been no curiosity. We talked about the role of diagnosis in driving this historical approach, in our experience, answering the question 'what are you experiencing?' Becomes translated into diagnostic categorising. We shared examples from our own experiences of when stereotypical psychotic experiences are enquired about through closed questioning, which has proved dangerous when our experiences have been undetected as they have not fitted within these particular categories. We therefore felt there needs to be a curiosity from staff, asking open questions and a sensitivity to the language people are using, taking time to find out about their experiences. We weren't surprised when on several occasions throughout the transcripts, the question of 'what is psychosis' arose, and we thought that there is a degree of inevitability when people's experiences do not fit into diagnostic categories and stereotypical symptoms.

In thinking more broadly about staff team approaches to working with psychosis, we reflected on our experiences of hearing the message from staff of 'you are wrong' (i.e. that sensory perceptions or beliefs are not based within a shared reality). We shared our experiences of finding this as a pivotal moment in the recovery process and one which can feel immensely damaging and depressing, bringing with it, a sense of needing to question 'everything' and believing that staff have a better grasp of reality than we do.

We talked about psychosis as being a load-bearing experience; you can't remove it without causing a lot of collateral damage. In our experience, once psychosis has been 'revealed' in this way, there follows a depression that does not always get addressed. If there was a way of salvaging something from the experiences that was meaningful, perhaps it would not have been such a devastating loss. We talked about this moment of realisation as being a distinct point, when you start becoming part-time in two dimensions. We felt that staff are often keen for this to happen but do not acknowledge the trauma; at this point, there is also a need to start taking responsibility for what happened when you were psychotic.

Psychosis Can Be a Meaningful Life Experience

As we observed the different repertoires around how psychosis can be a meaningful life experience, we spent some time discussing our own understandings of meaning and meaningfulness and comparing these to the transcripts. There was some discrepancy between our concept of meaning and that expressed by staff. We felt that staff talked around the idea of meaning, and we wondered whether they didn't fully understand the question, whether they didn't want to or were cautious of imposing their own meaning onto someone's experience of psychosis.

Within the transcripts, there were discussions around the notion of trauma, which we felt came the closest to making an interpretation of meaning. This led to a discussion between us of experiences of accessing mental health services and feeling as if staff have been desperately trying to find the trauma, in order to understand why we have experienced the psychosis. We reflected that an attempt to find meaning can get translated into trying to find a cause, which we felt were different things.

Extract 3: Staff Focus Group C

```
Nicky    '...we go in with the idea that how you are now will make

         sense to us if we can get enough information about what

         you've been through...'
```

(C: 255–257)

We agreed on the difficulty with trying to describe and interpret an experience that isn't something that happens through words. We consider psychosis to be an experience that is beyond words; it is images and sensory experiences, a bit like 'a waking dream', speaking through metaphor. In relation to psychosis and meaningfulness, we consider the experience of psychosis itself, to be like an 'explosion of meaning' where meaning and significance can be found everywhere in seemingly meaningless places, for example car number plates. In our experience of accessing mental health services, the meaning can get lost when professionals talk without the service user present. We felt that this can be a loss as the language used by service user is a means of communication that is important to them and represents a useful opportunity for staff to connect.

Reading the transcripts made us reflect on the broader society within which EI services are situated. We wondered whether it is the experience of psychosis that's the problem and or lack of social resources to allow a person to go through it. We thought about the social model of disability (Oliver, 1983); considering how psychosis might be socially constructed because society is not resourced to allow a person to go through a psychotic experience. Within society, there seem to be kinds of meaning people are allowed to give their experience and psychosis breaches those boundaries; i.e., there are certain things you're not allowed to believe if a fundamental belief of our culture is that these things don't exist.

In considering our differing understandings of psychosis, we wondered whether staff would view working with the content of psychosis as outside of their remit, perhaps more in the remit of psychology, and whether this accounted for the emphasis on providing psychosocial interventions, evident within the transcripts. We thought that it might be difficult for staff to talk about meanings; they may feel wary of making things worse, it may feel scary, and staff may feel judged by their peers. We wondered whether a mentoring relationship between staff and people with lived experience of psychosis might feel helpful, a way to 'check out' ideas, helping contextualise the experience and supporting navigation through it. At the same time, we acknowledged that the professional approach to working with psychosis is to minimise distress and as such considering the content of psychosis may not be aligned with this approach. We observed that there seemed to be a theme in this repertoire around a 'need for speed' of interventions which we thought might determine the ways in which meaning is understood or put aside, looking for ways to minimise risk.

We acknowledged that some of our ideas for exploring psychosis would mean working over a lifetime; our feelings were that once you accept what it has come to teach you, once you are engaging with the experience, it may resolve and dissipate; if left unresolved, it may return.

Though we felt it might be important to allow a person to explore the meaning of their psychosis, we talked from our own experiences of how it can be very difficult to find balance between going through psychosis and staying connected to the 'real world' (such as by maintaining work, relationships, eating, drinking, sleeping). We discussed a need to find some 'point of departure' from the experience, and how someone working at a level of meaningfulness might need to come back for their relationships. We also spoke about how it can be particularly difficult for friends and family members to understand and bear with a person's need to go through it. When at times the psychotic world may be appealing and seductive, we agreed that a balance needs to be found between respecting the experiences and their meanings and respecting relationships. In our experiences, it was meaningful relationships which supported us to re-engage with parts of the 'real world'.

Service Priorities

We thought the staff seemed to be conscious of how service priorities were related to a constrained environment which directed them to work in particular ways, painting a picture of a constrained service. Through reading the transcripts, we had a sense of how impossible it is from their perspective as staff to get the understanding you (as someone experiencing psychosis) want them to have. It appeared that the staff's main focus seemed to be working on reducing distress.

Extract 4: Staff Focus Group B

```
Julia    '…services are set up to focus on the degree of the

         illness rather than the nature of the illness, which

         then pushes us toward medication which then makes the

         meaning of a lesser importance…'
```

(B: 273–277)

We reflected that, if they've never experienced psychosis themselves, it might appear that the experience is always distressing. From the language used in the transcripts, we could see the staff were straining to find the best way to help, though we wondered whether if someone has not had the experience themselves, then there is a limited language and way of understanding. We thought that staff might only see suffering because this is why people with psychosis end up accessing mental health services, so it must look as if the two equate.

We felt empathy for the staff, feeling the pressure they are under. The red tape feels very real and staff are not able to escape the boxes that have been put in place by service constraints. The comment in the transcript around 'just having the time to be alongside someone' was felt appropriate, and from our experience, we understand that sometimes that is all you can do. However, we thought that if staff feel they do not have time to work in this way, it must be distressing for them.

Our overall impression of the EI services spoken about by staff was positive; this made us reflect that there might be a 'culture shock' for those people who transition to mainstream mental health services. Though we have not received EI services, we are familiar with mainstream mental health services and fear that the 'everyday' language used in EI teams may leave people unprepared for what may be to come. We fear they will not have the linguistic tools to be able to negotiate psychiatric settings and sadly felt that it may not prepare people for 'sub-standard care'.

Reflections on the Process of Involvement in the Project

Claire

On a personal level, it felt important to me to include the perspective of people with lived experience, in the research process. Within my clinical work, I aimed to promote opportunities for service receiver co-production at strategic levels, and therefore involvement on my doctoral research project was a natural fit with this way of working. However, once I had decided that involvement was going to be a key component of the research, I was uncertain of where to begin, mindful that involvement should be about making a valuable contribution to the research, rather than a tokenistic gesture.

I met Ben and Ashley through a local collective of people who have an interest in and/or experience of psychosis. As Ben and Ashley had been kind enough to volunteer their time, I wanted to keep the options open for them to be as involved as much or as little as they wanted. This openness also brought with it a level of anxiety as I wondered about roles and expectations, the idea of representation and how we were each defining our positions in relation to the research. It was helpful and reassuring that Ben and Ashely were open to talking these anxieties through together. As I described the concept of the research, we initially agreed to meet to provide a space in which I could reflect on my experiences as I progress with the research. This idea evolved to us reflecting on the data together.

Prior to conducting the focus groups, I was concerned that some of the content might feel upsetting to hear from the perspective of people who have received mental health services. However, I reflected on this concern as perhaps indicative of a level of paternalism between those providing and those receiving mental health services.

Meeting regularly with Ben and Ashley to read through the transcripts together has been an invigorating experience. I am grateful for their patience, enthusiasm and willingness to allow the data analysis process to evolve. Aware that I had not adopted a formal recruitment process, I hadn't anticipated that our conversations might provide further data. This presented a dilemma as to how to include this content; if the words of staff are included and those of people with lived experience are not, might this reflect power imbalances more generally. Therefore, collaborating on this chapter together has allowed us to both share our discussions and reflect on the experience overall.

Ashley

I first came into contact with Claire through an email from the Bridge Collective advertising an opportunity to get involved with a research project looking at the question of meaningfulness in psychosis. As someone who has experienced psychosis and been diagnosed with schizophrenia, I was interested in the project's attempt to talk about the meaningfulness of these experiences which tend to be written off as irrational nonsense. My own experience of psychosis was an explosion of meaning during which everything becomes significant and in need of decoding. So I was confused when I first read the transcripts of the EI teams' discussions of meaningfulness in their service users' experience of psychosis as they didn't seem to grasp the question. It was as if the meaning of the experience could only be understood in a linear sense of cause and effect, looking for triggers and life experiences that might lie behind the symptoms. This gap between my own experience of a plenitude of meaningfulness and the research findings became the start of a rich and wide-ranging conversation between the three research participants which went beyond the original brief of looking for discursive themes in the transcripts. The research gave me a rare opportunity to listen in on the way mental health workers talk about their service users' experiences, and I was struck by a sense of these people struggling to do the best they can with diminishing resources and under difficult conditions. However, there seemed to be a glass wall between those who work in mental health support and those they are trying to help and support. The conversations between the staff were complex and varied, launching off from the points we found in the transcripts to speculate on the context for those conversations and ways that might shift the conversation towards a shared language. This became a real opportunity to voice our own experiences in the light of the ideas raised by the EI teams.

Ben

I first heard about Early Intervention a couple of years after my first full-blown psychotic episode. It was a very new concept at the time, and I remember thinking how much benefit I could have gained if something like it had been available when I was first showing signs as a teenager. I was immediately sold on the idea, because Early Intervention had got to be better than the more traditional 'Fashionably Late Intervention' that I had experienced. Unfortunately, whenever I saw reports on it, there was always seemed to be an emphasis on handing out medication, and whilst I could see how people might view this as being proactive, I could only feel disappointed that such a great concept was being squandered with a narrow approach. Disappointment tends to lead to disengagement, and for many years I stopped paying any attention to what was happening in Early Intervention, focusing instead on solving the puzzle that my own psychosis had presented me with.

Of course, whilst first impressions are informative, they are not always wholly accurate. So when Claire asked for involvement from people with lived experience of psychosis, that same enthusiasm for a great concept combined with curiosity for how the field had developed since the early 2000s, and I agreed to read and comment upon interview transcripts from three different Early Intervention teams. I'm glad I did.

The teams I discovered through the transcripts were quite unlike the ones I had built in my imagination. They were actively averse to pushing medication and they were filled with doubt, both qualities I felt much more comfortable with. Having filled out many care plans which ended up gathering dust until the next time one needed filling out, I could thoroughly appreciate the unanimous desire to be rid of all the bureaucratic nonsense. They were all saying so many of the right things, with the right intention, that it almost felt rude to critique and comment upon what they had to say.

However, up and down this country, there are people who have never experienced psychosis, defining and interpreting the psychoses in other people. They use specialised forms of language that are both alien and alienating, whilst simultaneously assuming another's language is 'symptomatic'. Reading through the transcripts, I could not help but be forcefully reminded how often those of us with lived experience have been excluded from the conversation, talked about and interpreted via models that can reduce a meaningful communication to the status of a sound effect. That feeling of being one step removed from the action, of being wrong about everything and of being a 'them'.

To be invited to the conversation, to have that say, to have the right to critique and interpret, should never have been considered revolutionary, and yet at the same time, it still seems remarkable. The way that in each of the transcripts there was a straining at the limits of professional language, that there was so much angst noticeable when certain terms and terminology were used, clearly demonstrates the necessity for widening the conversation. It's nice to be part of the team, less so to be a service user.

Recommendations for Interprofessional Team Working

Our recommendations for interprofessional team working are arising from conversations which were stimulated by looking at the research data, making us reflect on differences between EI and traditional services.

We noted that sometimes communication across different professional disciplines can become tied up in their own theories (e.g. phenomenology vs biological determinism); we felt that the focus should remain on what is going to be most meaningful for the service user. Inviting the service user to meetings can therefore reduce the potential for interprofessional posturing. Also, this recognises having an experience of a condition as knowledge; even if it is not professional, it is still valuable. Teams should be mindful of outnumbering the person they are working with; if they are determined to include representatives from each profession, they should consider balancing this with the needs of the person.

In terms of language, we would recommend remaining mindful of some of the language used within mental health contexts which may appear confusing and paradoxical at best and offensive and frightening at worst. For example, 'positive symptoms of psychosis', implies that this is something 'good', rather than something 'additional', and 'co-morbid' might imply something 'deadly'.

We would recommend being open about unfamiliarity or awkwardness with particular terms which may seem politically incorrect (e.g. 'insight') as this may produce an opportunity for discussion. From our experiences, we have also sadly become aware that it is possible to hide stigmatising attitudes behind politically correct language, and we would recommend teams remain mindful of this.

Summary

Critical discursive psychology as a rapidly developing field remains largely within the realms of 'experts'. However, if this approach is to remain relevant to healthcare research, service user involvement is key. We hope that this study has demonstrated that it is possible to involve people who have received services in a helpful and meaningful way. By offering a third perspective as experts by experience (in addition to researcher and participant), further data have been produced which might indicate opportunity for developing this methodology.

Tips for doing research
Consider opportunities for involvement across all stages of the research process from concept, design, data collection, analysis and dissemination. Remain reflective throughout the process, is involvement going to be meaningful? Be transparent about roles, expectations and language (i.e. service user, expert-by-experience, co-researcher etc.). Remember it is better to start somewhere and include involvement at some level than none at all.

References

Bell, K. (2010). Cancer survivorship, mortality and lifestyle discourses on cancer prevention. *Sociology of Health & Illness, 32,* 349–364.

Billig, M., Condor, S., Edwards, D., Gane, M., Middleton, D., & Radley, A. (1988). *Ideological dilemmas: A social psychology of everyday thinking.* London: Sage.

Birchwood, M., Fowler, D., & Jackson, C. (Eds.). (2000). *Early intervention in psychosis: A guide to concepts, evidence and interventions.* Chichester: Wiley.

Boyle, M. (2002). *Schizophrenia—A scientific delusion?* (2nd ed.). Hove: Routledge.

Cooke, A. (Ed.). (2015). *Understanding psychosis and schizophrenia: Why people sometimes hear voices, believe things that others find strange or appear out of touch with reality, and what can help.* Leicester: British Psychological Society.

Davies, B., & Harré, R. (1990). Positioning: The discursive production of selves. *Journal for the Theory of Social Behaviour, 20*(1), 43–63.

Edley, N. (2001). Analyzing masculinity: Interpretative repertoires, ideological dilemmas and subject positions. In M. Wetherell, S. Taylor, & S. J. Yates (Eds.), *Discourse as data: A guide for analysis.* London: Sage.

Kelleher, I., Jenner, J. A., & Cannon, M. (2010). Psychotic symptoms in the general population—An evolutionary perspective. *British Journal of Psychiatry, 197*(3), 167–169. https://doi.org/10.1192/bjp.bp.109.076018.

Longden, E., (2013, August 7). *Eleanor Logden: The voices in my head* [video file]. Retrieved from https://www.ted.com/talks/eleanor_longden_the_voices_in_my_head/transcript, on 15 January 2017.

National Institute for Health Research. (2018). NETSCC's PPI framework and activity plan 2015–18. NIHR (downloaded from www.nihr.ac.uk. 4 June 2018).

Oliver, M. (1983). *Social work with disabled people*. Basingstoke: Macmillan.

Potter, J., & Wetherell, M. (1987). *Discourse and social psychology: Beyond attitudes and behaviour*. London: Sage.

Read, J., Mosher, L., & Bentall, R. (2004). *Models of madness: Psychological, social and biological approaches to schizophrenia*. Hove: Brunner-Routledge.

Roberts, G. (2000). Narrative and severe mental illness: What place do stories have in an evidence-based world? *Advances in Psychiatric Treatment, 6*(6): 432–441.

Roberts, G. (2006). Understanding madness. In G. Roberts, S. Davenport, F. Holloway, & T. Tattan (Eds.), *Enabling recovery: The principles and practice of rehabilitation psychiatry* (pp. 93–111). London: Royal College of Psychiatrists.

Taylor, S. (2013). *What is discourse analysis?* London: Bloomsbury.

Wetherell, M. (1998). Positioning and interpretative repertoires: Conversation analysis and post-structuralism in dialogue. *Discourse and Society, 9*(3), 387–412.

Williams, P. (2012, August 2) *Brain disease or existential crisis?* https://www.madinamerica.com/2012/08/op-ed-schizophreniapsychosis-brain-disease-or-existential-crisis/. Accessed 15 January 2017.

Part V

Interventions—Supporting Teamwork in Mental Health Care

14

Using Joint Conversation Analysis Between Clinicians and Researchers: Developing Reflexivity in Community Mental Health Teams

Cordet Smart, Holly Reed, Madeleine Tremblett and Nancy Froomberg

Introduction

Conversation Analysis and its extension Discursive Psychology (CA/DP) is used by researchers who have studied and trained in how to analyse conversation in this very specific manner (see Chapter 2). The growing literature on DP/CA means that it has become a complex field for the non-specialist to negotiate. Conversation Analysis (CA) risks losing its impact if it becomes too specialist for practitioners to understand and

C. Smart (✉) · H. Reed · M. Tremblett · N. Froomberg
School of Psychology, University of Plymouth, Plymouth, UK
e-mail: cordet.smart@plymouth.ac.uk

H. Reed
e-mail: holly.reed@students.plymouth.ac.uk

M. Tremblett
e-mail: madeleine.tremblett@plymouth.ac.uk

N. Froomberg
e-mail: nancy.froomberg@plymouth.ac.uk

© The Author(s) 2018
C. Smart and T. Auburn (eds.), *Interprofessional Care and Mental Health*,
The Language of Mental Health, https://doi.org/10.1007/978-3-319-98228-1_14

use themselves (see Chapter 3), yet its particular contribution comes from its unique way of exploring language. Therefore, as part of the *MDTsInAction* project, we wished to consider how we could make a DP/CA approach more participatory. This would enable us to:

- offer something back to our participants in terms of continuing professional development (CPD);
- consider how to ensure that the analysis reflects staff priorities; and
- develop an approach to DP/CA analysis that enables non-specialists to be involved in the analysis.

To achieve these aims, we included what we termed 'joint analysis' sessions within the research design. We defined 'joint analysis' as sessions where members of the research team, participants and other stakeholders—such as service users and carers—come together to analyse the team's data.

Data Groups

Data groups are a forum that qualitative researchers commonly use to explore data. They involve researchers bringing data, listening to data, analysing individually, and then discussing the analysis. Our own research group CARP (Conversation Analysis Research at Plymouth) has now been running for over 12 years, while perhaps the most famous one in CA is DARG (Discourse Analysis Research Group), which runs from Loughborough University (Edwards, 2012). Transcripts and their audio couterparts are discussed in detail with each member bringing their own expertise in applying CA principles to the target data. It is an opportunity for peer review of analytical interpretations and to this extent they enhance the plausibility of the analysis.

During a standard CARP session, the group will meet for around an hour and a half. One member of the group will bring some data from their current research project. These often will be short extracts of longer transcripts worked up using Jeffersonian transcription conventions. The group will listen to the extracts and together check for transcription errors and engage in analysis. There follows a round-table discussion of the data extract during which members talk through their own understanding of the talk using CA/DP principles (turn-taking, sequence organisation, repair) to dissect its social organisation (see Chapter 2 for some worked examples). Throughout the session, we remind each other to focus on the detail, to consider what else could have been said—why this phrase? Why was that said here? What comes next? What is the function of a phrase? Different techniques can be employed:

1. Presenting data and proposed CA interpretations to the group and the group discussing to what extent they agree.
2. Presenting data without context to explore applications of CA.
3. Presenting data with professional labels removed to explore the effects of these on reading the data.
4. Asking co-analysts for their opinions about what a data excerpt represents.
5. Clarification on transcription.
6. 'Device spotting'—practice in identifying known phenomena in the data such as types of repair.

Data groups enable the continued discussion and refinement of CA understandings of data for academics and provide an excellent educational context for students of CA (see Chapter 1). For example, Smart and Denman (2017) explored the challenges within a research supervision context of applying a Conversation Analytic approach to the development of a clinical doctorate which focused on family discussions of autism. In their chapter, they discuss how attendance at analysis sessions enabled the student (KD) to increase her confidence in CA. This included the opportunity to listen to more experienced analysts, as well as having to voice her own comment on the data. KD discusses the challenges that she experienced in this context of separating out clinical interpretations from conversation analytic ones and having to 'suspend' a more clinically interpretative way of thinking in order to focus on the talk at a turn-by-turn level.

Others have also recognised the importance of engaging in group research processes for students, as more valuable than attempting to learn through 'methodological manuals' (Frankham et al., 2014). Mostly, these research groups include only researchers or academics. It is unusual to include those outside of academic contexts.

Joint Analysis

We envisioned that 'joint analysis' groups would be organised in a similar way to CARP data sessions. We planned to include participants from the research and at least one researcher. Our 'joint analysis' compliments the increasing Public and Patient Involvement (PPI) requirements in healthcare contexts, which proposes those who use services should be consulted and involved throughout advancing healthcare services (Baxter, Thorne, & Mitchell, 2001; Millar, Chambers, & Giles, 2015; NICE, 2011). As discussed in Chapter 3, involvement in the *MDTsInAction* research problem was related to both service user and clinician involvement. Joint analysis enabled us to challenge gaps in understanding between academic research and clinical staff, increasing the credibility of real-world applications. It enhanced relationships between the research team and clinicians enabling ongoing communications so that we could hear how the research continued to influence practice, and teams could ask questions of the research.

Participant involvement is a concern not only of healthcare research, but also in qualitative research generally. Joint analysis is less common in Conversation Analytic research, and we struggled to find examples. However, there are examples from the fields of Interpretative Phenomenological Analysis (IPA) and narrative analysis. For example, Phoenix et al. (2016) explored how multiple interpretations could be developed of the same transcripts by including analysts from different philosophical underpinnings (psychoanalysis, thematic research, narrative, IPA and discourse, different cultural backgrounds, genders and ethnicities, and experiences of the focal topic). Unlocking these multiple possible explanations and understandings of people, they argued, enabled increased confidence in the research, and an 'opening up' of thinking for those participating. This complemented the 'multiple lens' approach of narrative analysis where sense-making is explored. Joint analysis within interprofessional groups might also ensure that the perspectives of different professionals are included in line with an interprofessional working approach. The analysis can then become multi-layered, providing mutual learning opportunities clinicians attending and researchers. Other authors have highlighted more directly the benefits of including service users in healthcare research. For example, Mjøsund et al. (2017) reported their own experiences with an IPA study, where a trained qualitative researcher worked with a group of non-researchers who had experienced mental health services. They found that inclusion of service users within the analysis significantly improved the nuance and the meaning that it was possible to apply to the findings. Further, this seemed to enhance the interpretative element of IPA. In another example, Sweeney, Greenwood, Williams, Wykes, and Rose (2013) included service users in a data analysis session. They used what they termed as a multiple coding technique, where each individual person conducted analysis of the transcripts on their own, and then came together to analyse them, reflecting on how they had developed the codes and examining where there were similarities and differences. The authors reported that this worked well in enhancing the interpretative element of the analytic approach, which is central to IPA. All of these authors note how the involvement of multiple perspectives seemed central to increasing confidence in terms of how the data analysis groups work.

How to organise a joint analysis group where the primary focus is on CA is perhaps less clear, in part because CA has developed a unique technical vocabulary. We reasoned that even without specialist knowledge, it would be a useful forum to test whether our interpretations made sense beyond our tight CA group. So we attempted in this study to follow a CA approach to data groups, despite not everyone having expertise. There was limited time, which meant that we had to be very clear in terms of what we wanted from clinicians. Our joint analysis sessions included clinicians—our participants—but unfortunately not service users or carers. The joint analysis was designed to involve our participants themselves in parts of the research other than being observed and recorded. Sometimes conversations focused on clinical implications rather than the organisation of talk, but this was also part of the benefit. The session provided new learning about the transcripts developed through group discussion, and new learning for clinicians in terms of the approach. We were able to add insight from those who were present in the original recording. Further, we explored with clinicians the possible practices that we had initially identified as relevant to the conduct and outcomes of the team meetings. We were mindful that this meant that some of the more technical terms of CA needed simplification to ensure that the data analysis was accessible by all of those present. This was not to 'water down' CA, but to enable it to be positioned within meaningful discourse for larger audiences. For example, in Chapter 11, we explored advocacy, including how experiences of service users are represented when they are not present. We identified how direct and indirect reported speech is relevant. However, the meanings of some of these ideas were not really obvious for practitioners until we explored this with them. Clinicians identified how these practices fitted with them 'doing' advocacy. Joining together practices of talking with the concept of advocacy produced more clinically meaningful interpretations.

Joint analysis, then, extends the notion of a data group to something that works quite differently. Additional features to data groups include:

1. Methodological application: The analysis group is not solely about the validation of methodological application,
   a. Methods can be questioned,
   b. Relevance to real-world contexts foregrounded;
2. Context outside of the immediate interaction can be considered;
3. Transcription: Can be checked directly with participants;
4. Clinician /non-specialist learning: Clinicians can learn a different way of understanding their interactions (it is likely that clinicians would be more keen for this than service users or some other stakeholders);
5. Joint reflection: Through combining new and different ways of thinking, new perspectives can emerge.

Project Overview

The process that we followed in engaging our research participants was broken down into different 'stages' of joint analysis. The orientation of the chapter is to report our learning about this process—what worked and what did not, constantly reflecting on what the real outcome or benefit of this approach was both for clinicians and for the development of the research. After setting out the protocol that we used for joint analysis, examples of two different joint analysis sessions are discussed. Within these examples, we aim to reveal something of the evolutionary nature of these sessions as they occurred through our research programme; the importance of careful presentation of data so that it is not too critical or uncomfortable for participants, and how clarifications in wording and speakers were obtained. We discuss how we increased the accessibility of CA for clinicians. Finally, we reflect on the particular process of joint analysis used, with recommendations for future approaches in this area. We also briefly discuss how these sessions were particularly relevant in signposting how best to organise the subsequent training sessions.

Stages of Joint Analysis

Stage 1: Arranging Sessions

Organising sessions was tricky. Reconnecting with teams following data collection was the first challenge encountered. In some cases, due to the availability of the researchers or the team, this was 6 months to 1 year following data collection. For those teams where the gap was shorter (1–3 months), it was generally easier to continue to promote engagement. This is an important consideration for larger scale research projects where there may be longer time periods involved.

A second consideration related to time and location. Generally, we found that trying to align joint analysis sessions with CPD sessions that the teams were already holding, or following meetings when multiple staff were already present, was also facilitative.

Other difficulties were around clinicians' levels of understanding of the expectations of these sessions and their benefits. Most had not engaged in qualitative analysis before and none had engaged in a joint analysis session. Within this preliminary programme of research, part of the process was to develop a protocol for conducting joint analysis, so it was difficult to pre-specify what this might be. For future studies, it is suggested that information be sent at the point of re-initiating contact, specifying this protocol for joint analysis, and that clinicians need have no prior knowledge to be involved.

Stage 2: Data Preparation

A considerable amount of data preparation was required. Clinician availability dictated that sessions were either 1 or 1.5 hours. A list of aims were developed prior to each session, for example, to analyse a transcript and compare with the research team's analysis, or to examine practices that confused researchers.

Once the aims were identified, data was transcribed orthographically and appropriate extracts were selected and transcribed using Jeffersonian transcription conventions. A balance had to be struck between not analysing the data too much in advance and ensuring each selection was relevant. We listened to large amounts of data and discussed the themes present including how this new data fitted with prior data analysis. We then identified extracts that seemed 'typical' of particular phenomena. Decisions were taken in accordance with the predetermined aims, but these also developed iteratively as we listened to more of the data. We sought to ensure that we could find interesting extracts that were relevant to clinical practice and the interests of teams.

Stage 3: Face-to-Face Discussion

We introduced ourselves and brought to sessions a short power point just reminding people of the research aims and explaining that CA is about looking at the different actions of utterances in talk. We provided 3 handouts—one a summary of Jeffersonian transcription symbols, quick and dirty CA, and the focal extract (See Appendix A for an example). For the earlier sessions, we took three extracts, but it was soon apparent that there was only time for one. The exact approach varied, but we aimed for 10–15 minutes introduction, 5–10 minutes listening, 30 minutes discussion and 5 minutes conclusions/wrapping up. Sessions were either audio recorded or detailed notes were taken.

Stage 4: Summary and Feedback

After the session, notes were collated and sent to the groups for their comments. Additional reflections were then included and added to the notes. These notes informed the analysis so that comments could be drawn on when writing up and also informed subsequent training sessions.

Stage 5: Feedback into Final Topic Focus

Feedback from the sessions was discussed in *MDTsInAction* research programme meetings in order to influence the overall direction of the research and was used to guide and shape the analysis. For example, to refine the focus of a collection, or to discard something that was less clinically relevant.

Two examples are presented here from the joint analysis sessions that were run, in order to illustrate the way that the process worked.

Example 1: Community Learning Disability Team

People Present
This session involved 3 members of the research team, the Principal Investigator (CS), Research Assistant (HR) and a PhD student (MT). From the MDT, a Student Nurse, a Community nurse, a Senior nurse (team leader) and a Clinical Psychologist attended.

Aims of the Session
We took in 3 broad aims:

- To check out some of our ideas
- To do some analysis together
- To gain feedback around what is most interesting and relevant for clinicians.

Structure

In order to set the scene of the meeting, we began by reminding participants of the main research aims. We then discussed the main aims of the study, to examine teams in terms of:

- Intra-Team function
- Organisational factors—structure of the meetings, location, etc.
- Clinical action of the meetings.

We then outlined the main principles of CA, using four key concepts:

- Sequence organisation and Adjacency pairs
- Epistemics
- Repair
- Turn-taking.

We introduced some of our findings from other research and then started to run a data session in the way that CARP and other analysis groups do. This would normally involve introducing an extract of talk, playing the recording, examining the detailed transcript and then discussing it.

Summary

In the actual event, we discussed a little of the overview of the research, but there was not quite enough time to include all its different dimensions. We chose to go with the direction of clinicians. Clinicians wanted to have space to discuss what it was like to be recorded, and feeling self-conscious about the recordings. They had slightly different perceptions and it was really helpful to hear that they experienced being aware of the presence of the tape for quite a long time, and that then this awareness faded out, which they estimated took around 30 minutes. Extract 1 was used in the session:

Extract 1: Presenting Patient Experiences (an Example of an Extract Used in One Session)

(CPs: Clinical Psychologist; CMN: Community Nurse; SLT: Senior Team Leader)

```
1  CPs:    Oh she's lo:vely=

2  CMN:    (she is)

3  CPs:    =she's s:o: lovely

4  CMN:    but she's quite >she's a vulnerable lady

5          She when< she she'll take herself off on

6          the train to (place)< and then

7  CPs:    she's quite often at (place) train station

8          'aving=a cup of t:ea↓

9  SLT:    yeah↓ cause her husband's off doing his e:r

10 CPs:    °cleaning°

11 CMN:    Yea:h

12 CPs:    °(whereas she used to stay in)° alot

13 CPs:    we did some really brief

14         CBT with her it was quite effective

15         °actually°

16 CPs:    I don't think you could unpick it now

17         sands of time stuff probably ye:s
```

Response to the Extract

In this extract, clinicians did not seem self-conscious—they spoke confidently and focused on the service user under discussion. This contrasted with clinician's descriptions of themselves as being quieter and very distracted. The extract was only 5 minutes into the meeting, so it seemed that the distraction by the tape was less persistent than was claimed.

A second theme was the keenness of the participants to understand how the dynamics of the team worked—clinicians wanted to know from us what had best worked or not, and what we were able to identify. It was difficult to identify these concerns within this one extract. Clinicians were also interested in who spoke most, and commented on how well the service user being discussed was known to the team. We decided that this could also be evidenced in statements such as 'she's sooo lovely' (line 1). This seemed to demonstrate a form of personal knowledge.

A particular challenge was that as this was the first session, we had hoped as researchers to focus the research on the data, and what clinicians felt around the data, but clinicians were more interested in discussing the general context. This information was later helpful in terms of contextualising the information, and working out which parts were more interesting. For example, it encouraged us to consider relationships between participants more, which interested the team (see Chapters 5–7). From this session, we developed principles for subsequent joint analysis sessions, which included:

- To have more focused aims around the potential outcomes;
- To reduce the introduction to ensure that there was enough time for data analysis; and
- To be accepting of the different perspectives of clinicians.

Example 2: A Rural Community Learning Disability Team

People Present
The session included the PI (CS), an Assistant Psychologist, a Community Liaison Nurse, a Speech and Language Therapist, a Senior Clinical Psychologist, a Learning Disability Nurse and a Physiotherapist.

Aims

This was the fourth joint analysis session held during the research programme, and based on prior learning, we refined the aims of the session to make them much more specific to the analysis of the team being studied. This seemed to enable to clinicians to be more focused and engaged.

- To briefly introduce the overall research programme structure
- To play and read the data
- Think about the data
- Reflect on central themes including:

  - Advocacy
  - Compassion
  - Interprofessional working.

The themes were developed in a discussion between three researchers (HR, BS, CS) prior to the joint analysis session, based on orthographic transcription of the data. Researchers identified key themes that had emerged as interesting and relevant, in the light of the prior research foci: the functioning of teams, their organisational situated nature and clinical practice. These themes seemed particularly relevant to the collections that were being developed from analysis of the data from this team. A typical extract was identified and transcribed in Jeffersonian format in order to explore these themes, and to explore how clinicians viewed the same extract (see Extract 2).

Structure

The session was booked for 1 hour, but ran over into 1.5 hours. We found that 1.5 hours was a good length of time for the session in order to ensure that there was enough time to discuss the data. The session began with a general introduction by the researcher and an overview of the main themes of the research programme. This seems to help clinicians to make sense of the ways that we are considering teams to operate.

We then discussed very briefly CA and the focus on language—three clinicians had some experience of this form of analysis in the past. In order to introduce the ideas briefly, we highlighted how we were going to focus on the details of conversation in order to be reflective on what processes were going on for individuals. This type of language seemed to enable clinicians to more easily make sense of the work to be done. Finally, we spent time discussing the selected extract.

Summary of Joint Analysis Session

Clinicians were keen to ask why the research team had selected the particular extract brought (Extract 2). However, the researcher explained that it might be more interesting first for them to present their thoughts and feelings related to the transcript, and then for us to discuss the rationale for selection. The extract focused on a discussion of a service user who felt that he was struggling to talk, and the different perspectives of the nursing home and his GP. This time we took a single, slightly longer extract.

Extract 2: Focal Extract Used for Joint Analysis in Example 2

SNP—Senior Practitioner and Chair; APs—Assistant Psychologist; OT Occupational Therapist; SLP—Speech and Language Therapist. Also present at the meeting: Assistant practitioner, Physiotherapist, Occupational therapist, Primary care learning disability nurse and Team administrator.

```
1   SNP      'kay .hh and then moving on t:o Dave

2            another referral from ↑Sam ↓Burrows↑

3   APs      (Shes off on sick leave)

4   SNP      she is .hhh

5   APs      ha ha

6   SNP      Uh ha this time for .hh SALT .hhh (.) ↑em:m

7            (and/but) this did make m:e ↓giggle (.) a

8            little bit hhh em (.) only because it's a

9            referral for Dave because Dave says that he

10           can't talk and his

11           throat hu:rts and he has been to the GP↓
```

```
12              but staffs=concerned that

13              Dave is ↑shouting↓

14   ???        hu ha ha ha

15              Hu ha

16              ha

17   SLP        [Can I:I

18   SNP        [and they are debating that this
19   SLP        I have worked before and he is alwa:ys .hh he

20              has quite often done that.

21              He has quite often said .hh

22              <I can't speak> and I think that is probably

23              because [>He doesn't want to<

24   ???              [Shouting

25   ???              [ah ha ha ha ha ha

26   ???              [I really feel that he is

27              just not being listened to

28   SLP              [He is either shouting or he

29              just doesn't want to £talk I think it's

30              sometimes a way of him saying I don't want to

31              talk to you

32   SNP        Yea, OK well maybe we'll just link in with Sam

33              Then and see what we can come up with

34   SLP        Sam does >add in a little bit more< (.)

35   SNP        Ok:ay↓
```

```
36   SLP      in an email

37            which say:s em

38            Dave >has a timetable< but=sta:ff (.) not (.)

39            Support(.)ing it >to be< us:ed

40            OK so it is like a communication=

41            =Dave is able to sign ↓but=staff ↓ca:n't

42            ↓sig:n back

43   SNP      Oh↓↓

44   SLP      That's staff skills ↑really, isn't it

45            [Is that em Acorn house

46   ???      [(?)

47   ???      Yea

48   SLP      and and Dave is saying that he can't

49            talk >°(because/and)

50            his throat hurts°< he has be:en to the GP

51            >I don't know what the outcome< was with the GP

52            em David is the la:st original↑ resident of the

53            home. He is shown feelings of being lost in

54            his own ho:me↓ There=has a lot of change

55            within the home (recently with staff) and

56            another resident who died

57            who ate meals with him.  Staff concerned

58            that David is shouting and invading pers:onal

59            space.hhh   He has autism↓ and anxiety↓↓~
```

```
60          and needs to be able to feel safe at home.~

61          So Denise Berry and Charlie Brown are

62          already involved

63   SNP    It's an ongoing problem ↑really↓
```

Not all of the clinicians present had been involved in a team meeting recording, nor involved in the extract presented. However, the senior nurse practitioner was present and as we can see from Extract 2 did most of the speaking. She expressed feeling anxious after hearing it, and we gave some time just to listen and not to comment on the transcript until people got used to hearing their voices. It was therefore important to introduce this delicately, the researcher explained that she had done a lot of self-listening, and we discussed how this could influence team processes and awareness.

The first discussion point was around how compassionate people could sound. The senior nurse practitioner asked about why there were downward arrows after her speech (lines 12, 10, 33 and 53). We discussed what this seemed to do, and how it seemed to bring 'compassion' into the conversation, a more sympathetic understanding seemed to be heard. It seemed to reflect the gravity of the situation.

There were discussions around how one practitioner (the speech and language practitioner) was able to steer another. For example, in line 44, where she comments 'that's skills stuff really, isn't it?', as if to direct more the nurse's telling of the story. This leads to a discussion of how different types of knowledge from different practitioners were able to complement each other. For example, the nurse's experiential knowledge of meeting the service user and discussing his needs with different people—his GP and staff at the nursing home; compared to the expert knowledge of the speech and language therapist, and her discussion of the skills needed by the service user and the care home.

The main emergent issue from the discussion was the challenges that the staff had experienced in advocating for the service user. There was a clear interpretation of his rationale for not talking—'Dave is able to sign, but staff can't sign back' (line 41–42); and a very sad explanation for how he might feel lonely in lines 52–57.

The joint analysis session enabled:

- Questioning and discussion around intonation made more obvious through the use of Jeffersonian transcription, such as downward arrows and intonation.
- Clarification of the relevance of the themes selected for clinical practice and development.

Key points that we took away for future sessions included:

- Future sessions should ideally be 1.5 hours as this enabled more time to look at the transcript.
- Clinicians enjoyed the listening and staged process of a brief introduction, time to comment on transcription, time to discuss intonation and summary of how this might work in the analysis and future meetings.
- Where possible it might be beneficial to run three sessions, one to check transcription, one to explore interesting phenomena and one to reflect on implications.

Summary

In summary, we attempted to run a series of joint analysis sessions where members of the teams whose voices we had recorded were involved in analysing some of the meetings that were the focus for the research. This form of joint analysis is perhaps unusual in CA and raises particular issues in terms of how the data is conceptualised—is it possible for us then to remove our assumptions and aim to try and reveal common sense. However, in practice, the input from clinicians enabled the credibility of the research to be developed in several ways. This included greater confidence that the analysis was focused on issues relevant to clinical practice which would subsequently be useful for clinical practice in real-world contexts.

Reflections on the Process of Joint Analysis

We attempted to 'formalise' a process of joint analysis here. We hoped to draw out, through our experiences, the barriers and facilitators to the approach, and to reflect a feasible way of engaging in participative designs that fit with contemporary approaches to research in health care (See Chapter 3's discussion of ethics). In some ways the process was problematic—time meant that a particular part of the analysis became the focus, and participants were not involved in orthographic transcription or selection of particular excerpts. This time constraint was overcome by running sessions in a similar way to academic analysis settings—bringing a transcript and analysing it. There were both advantages and disadvantages with this academic model.

An academic model of an analysis group allowed a clear and established approach to qualitative analysis to be drawn on within the joint analysis sessions. Therefore, clinicians had the opportunity to be involved in qualitative analysis of their own material. Thus through participation within the research process they could engage in continued professional development and update their skill set. It also enabled a clear model for researchers to use and confidence that this approach was not too different from everyday practice.

A second benefit of this process of joint analysis was that it became apparent how analysis in this way could facilitate clinicians with a particular form of reflexivity in their work. Reflexivity is a central concept in clinical practice (see Chapter 15). Importantly, this is about thinking through how practice works, and exploring how to improve it. There are a number of general models of reflective practice (e.g. Stedmon & Dallos, 2009), but it is also relevant to consider that within healthcare teams, different healthcare practitioners hold different models of reflexivity. Nevertheless, in order to enable reflexivity, a practitioner must in some way stand outside of a situation and look into it as an outsider. Listening to recorded team interactions and following these on the transcript were a very effective way for clinicians to take a reflective stance. Doing this as a team enabled a number of clinicians to mention some of the common cycles that the team engaged in, which could then be seen in the details of how people spoke.

However, this approach did also limit the engagement with the joint analysis sessions. For example, it might have been interesting and relevant for clinicians to have engaged in the process of developing the foci for analysis, and selecting extracts for more detailed study. This might have led to a greater proliferation of topics studied, particularly as the research team was composed of service users, carers, psychologists and one nurse, but other professions were not well represented. It also may have led to greater investment within the research.

The project also raises more general issues. In the introduction to this chapter, and in Chapter 3, we discussed how the specialist nature of CA can exclude non-specialists from the analysis. However, our experiences might imply that joint analysis is beneficial in terms of really enabling a 'fleshing out' of the context and greater confidence in the credibility of the work. The role of the researcher became one of facilitator rather than of direct leadership, of preparing the material, and laying it open to systematic thinking through. We did not always tape sessions—sometimes we did, and sometimes we just took notes. In some ways this took the pressure away from participants, enabling them to feel less observed, and more a part of the research process. In overview, the contributions were beneficial and allowed researchers to include humanised reflections on the CA interpretations and language that was used.

Implications for Interprofessional Working

As the sessions were conducted towards the end of the research project, we also took the opportunity to ask and think about implications of the project for staff training. One of the main themes that came through within the discussions with these joint analysis sessions was a desire to be trained in the methods (DP/CA), and a desire to be involved in the development of the project. Key learning that might enhance interprofessional working in mental health includes:

- Reflective practice in teams might be enhanced by recording and analysing team meetings.

- This might in particular be beneficial if facilitated by someone skilled in CA or DP, in order to facilitate understanding of the social organisation of the MDT meetings.
- Conceptualising teams as operating in different domains: interpersonal, organisational and clinical was helpful for professionals to separate out some of the complexities of team dynamics.
- Participating in joint analysis groups such as these was also helpful for clinicians to clarify and discuss the meanings of concepts central to clinical work such as: advocacy, interprofessional working and compassion.

Based on these joint analysis sessions, and the multiple research projects subsumed into this research programme, we have now piloted some of these ideas in the development of workshops, detailed further in the next chapter.

Appendix A—Handouts Used

(See, Table 14.1 and Fig. 14.1).

Table 14.1 Transcription symbols adapted from Jefferson (1984)

Transcription symbol	Meaning
(.)	Pause
=	'Latched' talk directly continued from the previous
:	Lengthening of a word
£	Smiley voice
Underlining	Emphasis in talk
↓	Downward intonation
↑	Upward intonation
(uncertainty)	Uncertainty in the accuracy of transcription
,	Slight upward intonation
.hhh	In-breath
hhh.	Out-breath
.	Final intonation
>rapid talk<	Fast speech
[overlap]	Start/end of overlapping speech
°quieter talk°	Talk noticeably quieter than surrounding talk
→	Line of interest

Quick and Dirty Conversation Analysis

- It is about thinking about how speech is delivered – for example the way that a sentence is constructed – not *what* is said, but *how* it is said;
- It is about how things are *received*: How people work together to move the conversation along.
- Some key concepts include:
  - Where there is 'trouble' within a conversation and this is corrected, or 'repaired'
  - How interruptions, upgrading a response (repeating it, for example), or laughter are able to demonstrate an 'action' such as agreement, disagreement or ultimately decision making.
- Through analysing text in this way, we are able to explore how particular features in a conversation are used or ignored.

Fig. 14.1 Handout used to introduce conversation analysis

References

Baxter, L., Thorne, T., & Mitchell, A. (2001). *Small voices big noises*. Exeter: Washington Singer Press. This report is also available from the INVOLVE website: www.invo.org.uk.

Edwards, D. (2012). Discursive and scientific psychology. *British Journal of Social Psychology, 51*(3), 425–435.

Frankham, J., Stronach, I., Bibi-Nawaz, S., Cahill, G., Cui, V., Dymoke, M., …, Mohd Khir, M. (2014). Deskilling data analysis: The virtues of dancing in the dark. *International Journal of Research & Method in Education, 37*(1), 87–100. https://doi.org/10.1080/1743727X.2013.795531.

Jefferson, G. (1984). On stepwise transition from talk about a trouble to inappropriately next-positioned matters. In J. M. Atkinson & J. C. Heritage (Eds.), *Structures of social action: Studies of conversation analysis* (pp. 191–222). Cambridge, UK: Cambridge University Press.

Millar, S., Chambers, M., & Giles, M. (2015). Service user involvement in mental health care: An evolutionary concept analysis. *Health Expectations*. https://doi.org/10.1111/hex.12353.

Mjøsund, N. H., Eriksson, M., Espnes, G. A., Haaland-Øverby, M., Jensen, S. L., Norheim, I., …, Vinje, H. F. (2017). Service user involvement enhanced the research quality in a study using interpretative phenomenological analysis—The power of multiple perspectives. *Journal of Advanced Nursing, 73*(1), 265–278.

NICE. (2011). *NICE CG136: Service user experience in adult mental health: Improving the experience of care for people using adult NHS mental health services*. London: NICE.

Phoenix, A., Brannen, J., Elliott, H., Smithson, J., Morris, P., Smart, C., …, Bauer, E. (2016, April). Group analysis in practice: Narrative approaches. *Forum Qualitative Sozialforschung/Forum: Qualitative Social Research*. https://doi.org/10.17169/fqs-17.2.2391.

Smart, C. A., & Denman, K. (2017). Student and supervisor experiences of learning and teaching conversation analysis and discursive psychology for autism spectrum disorder focused research: A reflective approach. In M. O'Reilly, J. Lester, & T. Muskett (Eds.), *A practical guide to social interaction research in autism spectrum disorders*. London: Palgrave Macmillan.

Stedmon, J., & Dallos, R. (2009). *Reflective practice in psychotherapy and counselling*. London: McGraw-Hill Education.

Sweeney, A., Greenwood, K. E., Williams, S., Wykes, T., & Rose, D. S. (2013). Hearing the voices of service user researchers in collaborative qualitative data analysis: The case for multiple coding. *Health Expectations, 16*(4), 89–99.

15

Training for Enhanced Team Performance in Mental Healthcare Contexts: A Workshop and Its Fit with Interprofessional Care

Cordet Smart, Holly Reed, Brajan Sztorc, Dominique Clancy and Emily Connolly

Introduction

A central aim of the *MDTsInAction* project was to ensure that our research would benefit staff, and ultimately, improve care for service users; the development of training workshops was central to this aim. Workshops combined principles from Conversation Analysis, interprofessional care and our findings. Working from a Conversation Analytic perspective, Liz Stokoe (2014) highlighted the problems with role-play as a training method,

C. Smart (✉) · H. Reed · B. Sztorc · D. Clancy · E. Connolly
School of Psychology, University of Plymouth, Plymouth, UK
e-mail: cordet.smart@plymouth.ac.uk

H. Reed
e-mail: holly.reed@students.plymouth.ac.uk

D. Clancy
e-mail: dominique.clancy@postgrad.plymouth.ac.uk

E. Connolly
e-mail: emily.connolly@plymouth.ac.uk

© The Author(s) 2018
C. Smart and T. Auburn (eds.), *Interprofessional Care and Mental Health*,
The Language of Mental Health, https://doi.org/10.1007/978-3-319-98228-1_15

arguing that simulated approaches can miss an understanding of how performances actually operate in practice. She argued that they are idealised versions of practice that do not reflect busy work contexts. Nevertheless, in practice in interprofessional education (IPE) simulations are often used for ethical reasons. Our workshops tried to balance these influences and:

1. Focused on the interprofessional elements of MDT interactions;
2. Presented example of logistical challenges in MDTs;
3. Used actual examples of clinical practice;
4. Were based on actual clinical events relevant to everyday contexts;
5. Focused on enhancing understanding of how interactions work; and
6. Promoted honest reflection on actual, rather than ideal clinical practice.

This chapter begins with an overview of training methods in interprofessional collaboration, drawing out key points relevant to the *MDTsInAction* workshops. It presents a critique of these approaches providing a rationale for training professionals within their professional environments. We then present how we used our research to develop a training programme. Our experiences of conducting two workshops will be elaborated, including an overview of the design of the workshops, how attendees experienced the workshops, and how they related this to their practice. Where other chapters have focused largely on interprofessional working (IPW), this chapter also reviews IPE. This is because more research has been undertaken in educational contexts that relates directly to developing training approaches.

Training for Interprofessional Working in Mental Health Contexts and Beyond: Interprofessional Education (IPE)

In 1974 Bernard Bandler described in detail the importance of mental health professionals working together. He discussed the overlap between professional expertise, and how social and organisational power and professional identity can compromise joint working. There have been a divergent trajectories in the development of interprofessional collaboration. On the one hand Interprofessional Education (IPE) is focused on the initial education and training of professionals, whereas Interprofessional Working IPW is focused on the practice of working and collaborating together and trying to fix or improve systems for those needing to work this way. The IPE movement is based on the assumption that training for IPW is best implemented at the educational level so that new professionals are better prepared, enabling values and training differences to be overcome (Pecukonis, Doyle, & Bliss, 2008). Much research on interprofessional collaboration has been conducted on IPE, in part related to the ease of access to educational as opposed to clinical contexts. In this chapter, for a rounded picture, we describe some recent developments in IPE and how they may dovetail with the practice of IPW. We describe two IPE initiatives: one initiative focused on teaching strategies that can be used in professional training programmes, the second focused on extra-curricular opportunities for in-training professionals.

Interprofessional Education Embedded Within Professional Training Programmes

Firstly, we discuss briefly some of the challenges inherent in teaching interprofessional collaboration that is embedded within educational programmes. Addressing these challenges has resulted in a proliferation of teaching methods. Questions have been raised as to whether training should be didactic, experiential, cooperative (across disciplines) or facilitated discussions. In taught environments, it is for a 'trainer' or 'teacher' to tell students about IPW and learning. Teaching might be done in groups considering issues such as how teams work together, process information together and what collaboration really is. In facilitated approaches, conversely, learning tends to be more problem based, where trainees and students are given a problem to solve together, facilitated by a workshop leader (Lindqvist & Reeves, 2007). These simulated experiences (Boet, Bould, Burn, & Reeves, 2014), it is argued, enable the greatest amount of hands-on learning, without negative consequences to service users. Within facilitated learning, issues are likely to emerge from engagement with the task, and any which do not arise during the session can be identified at the end of the session by the facilitator.

Boet et al. (2014) developed a list of principles that can be used to develop effective interprofessional learning:

1. Focus on the interprofessional—that is foreground interprofessional concerns;
2. Anticipate logistical challenges—when designing training between departments there can be issues of funding and relative responsibility.
3. Identifying interprofessional 'champions'—invested individuals who promote the inclusion of interprofessional learning in the curriculum.
4. Balance diversity with equity—that is try to have a balanced number of different professionals within the group, so that one profession does not dominate.
5. Develop scenarios that are relevant to all professionals.
6. Be mindful of 'sociological fidelity'—that is whether the simulated problem simply reproduces current hierarchies, or whether there is space to challenge and reform working practices into new, more collaborative methods.
7. The importance of pre-briefing—that is, setting the expectations for how the group will work.
8. The importance of debriefing, and the challenges of people feeling 'safe' enough to express feelings about their experiences.
9. Use of simulation to support the curriculum—that is use examples where IPW is central, such as ward rounds.
10. Focus the assessment on the team—so that the group clearly has to work together to achieve set outcomes.
11. Support those facilitating the sessions—this can be challenging and people might have to manage quite diverse approaches.
12. Use sessions as opportunities for research to develop the field.

While these guidelines are mainly targeted at simulated experiences for students, they have relevance in their ability to highlight the inherent issues of training those already engaged in interprofessional working. They also help in identifiying the criteria of validity within the *MDTsInAction* training project. For example, in our work some of these considerations were less of an issue; by directly engaging with practice, we were able to ensure that the discussions were relevant to practitioners. However, we had less control over who was able to attend.

Interprofessional Education: Extra-Curricular Opportunities

IPE is very relevant to professionals who are undertaking training. We present two examples here of IPE, drawn directly from initiatives currently operating within Plymouth University, UK. Trainee Clinical Psychologists involved with each programme present their perspectives on their involvement in these initiatives; these provide some insight into the ways that these initiatives have worked for the participants.

'Bridges'—A Student Led Group Operating Independently of the Educational Curriculum, Aiming to Build Bridges Between Different Professionals and Service Users

'Bridges' was established at Plymouth University in 2013 when a group of students from different disciplines (initially nursing, medicine and clinical psychology), inspired by an interdisciplinary staff conference, sought to create greater opportunities for interprofessional learning. Plymouth University provided the perfect forum for such a group, given its high proportion of health & social care courses, ranging from undergraduate programmes through to doctorate level qualifications. Although staff were enthusiastic to provide these opportunities, constraints such as timetabling, differing course demands and staff availability meant that opportunities for further learning were not easy to facilitate. Thus, students from various health and social care professions formed a steering group to devise a programme of events, which could fuel their own and others' appetites for greater exchange of experience and knowledge.

From the outset, a key component of the *Bridges* ethos was the importance of being a student-led initiative. A steering group was established to direct activities; however, to avoid the replication of traditional hierarchies typically found in multidisciplinary teams, roles within the group were flexible and subject to change dependent on academic commitments. Moreover, the group aimed to be led by the community of health and social care students at the University, with the objective of creating events reflecting their interests and ideas. Events have included annual conferences on relevant interprofessional topics (e.g. the context of austerity), clinical days (e.g. cardiac day, mental health day) and myth-busting sessions.

Throughout their studies, health and social care students typically engage in clinical placements. These placements frequently bring students into contact with other health and social care professionals, often when working as part of multidisciplinary teams. Early interactions and connections with other professions not only influence students' immediate clinical practice, but may also shape their opinions of, and interactions with, certain professions for the entirety of their careers. One annual *Bridges* event provided a forum to 'myth-bust' ideas about the roles of other health and social care professions, and to establish connections early in students' careers. Participants were invited to write any thoughts about professions including stereotypes and clichés, questions about their role or personal views. Following this initial exercise, the contents of each page were discussed with students from the named profession, with a view to myth-busting ideas and answering questions. Such an activity has the potential to spark anxiety and defensiveness in response to negative views about one's own profession. However, in participating alongside other health and social care professions, vulnerabilities were shared enabling individuals to feel safe to explore and question misperceptions. Whilst it is sometimes difficult to confront negative views about one's own profession, this process enabled participants to acknowledge these views, consider why they might be held, and reflect on how to take steps to change such views. In discussions, participants were often struck by how little they knew of other's professions and how challenges that were perceived as exclusive to their own profession were often in fact shared.

A pertinent theme raised in *Bridges* meetings was a shared frustration that opportunities to meet with other health and social care professions were very rare. Without time set aside for interprofessional learning across all health and social care professions, *Bridges* relies on students volunteering ideas and time. This is undoubtedly a challenge, particularly as interests from year to year may fluctuate and involvement may wane. On the other hand, it is perhaps a notable strength of *Bridges* that it operates outside of an assessed, educational context. This enables students to engage more freely with content and with reduced concerns of exposing a lack of knowledge. It is hoped that these opportunities for interaction increase students' awareness of, and solidarity with, other professionals encouraging them to return to clinical practice with an openness to others' experiences.

The unique feature of *Bridges* is that it is student led and so can contribute towards a creative regeneration of ideas. A key feature of the scheme is that strong 'Champions' are needed to ensure its continuation and development, but it has advantages in that students are able to negotiate its format and what they need from it.

Despite the numerous advantages of this programme, *Bridges* occurs before students graduate and there is no mechanism for ensuring that the learning gained on *Bridges* is maintained into their working practice. Further, it relies the implementation of 'safe' meetings with other students. It is difficult, therefore, for this simulated context to capture the actualities of IPW, and it seems likely a useful preparation, but does not train for actualities.

Schwartz Rounds—*A Way of Managing Emotional and Challenging Issues in Practice Together*

A second local initiative is the use of Schwartz Rounds in educational settings. Schwartz Rounds are an approach for groups of professionals to come together and manage difficult emotional experiences. This is an initiative that aims to promote compassionate care—that is care where professionals and service users are valued, and teams engage with IPW. Originally developed in the USA (called Schwartz Center Rounds),

Schwartz Rounds were part of the legacy of Kenneth Schwartz, a healthcare lawyer who, during treatment for lung cancer, observed variability in staff compassion towards him. He noted how the highly pressured hospital context can 'stifle inherent compassion and humanity' (Schwartz, 1995, p. 3). Schwartz Rounds aim to provide space for multidisciplinary staff to reflect upon their work in order to preserve the human connection in health care (Point of Care Foundation, 2015). Each Round lasts one hour, beginning with a panel of staff who present stories focused around a theme, such as 'a patient I will never forget'. The audience are then invited to join the discussion, guided by two facilitators who encourage focus on thoughts and feelings, as opposed to problem-solving.

Schwartz Rounds were piloted in the UK in 2009 by the Point of Care Foundation who continue to support over 150 organisations in running Rounds. Implementation of Schwartz Rounds into healthcare settings was recommended in the Francis Report, the outcome of an inquiry into Mid-Staffordshire Hospital where high patient death numbers were associated with neglect, preoccupation with targets and savings, and toxic and dysfunctional cultures (Francis, 2010, 2013). Schwartz Rounds were recommended as a cultural change mechanism because of their positive impact on IPW, compassionate care and staff well-being.

Research has found that attending Schwartz Rounds leads to improvements in staff well-being; reducing psychological distress, strengthening interdisciplinary working, reducing isolation, and increasing empathy and compassion to both staff and patients (e.g. Goodrich, 2011; Maben et al., 2017; Reed, Cullen, Gannon, Knight, & Todd, 2015; Robert et al., 2017). Causal mechanisms for change have been identified as the creation of countercultural space in which staff can tell stories, engage in self-disclosure and role-modelling vulnerability, experience emotional safety and containment, and find space for reflection and resonance (Maben et al., 2017). Through creating space to normalise emotions and promote interconnectedness, psychological withdrawal and dehumanisation of patients are likely to reduce and patient care improve (George, 2016).

Though Schwartz Rounds were developed for healthcare settings, their use has been extended to education contexts. This move is in support of nursing and medical professional bodies, who have stated that more needs to be done to prepare students and develop their resilience during training (Nursing and Midwifery Council [NMC], 2010; General Medical Council [GMC], 2015). It has been suggested that acculturation begins in medical school, whereby barriers to accessing support develop when role models do not normalise health access and stigma is propagated by the system (Hooper, Meakin & Jones, 2005; Roberts, Warner, & Trumpower, 2000). It is hoped that Rounds can impact on this acculturation, introducing reflective and multi-professional support sooner in training, fostering compassion, encouraging communication between professions and contributing to cultural change (Barker, Cornwell, & Gishen, 2016).

There is currently limited research exploring the impact of Schwartz Rounds in education, research is ongoing (e.g. at the University of Liverpool) and early results are promising. In an evaluation of the implementation of Schwartz Rounds into the medical curriculum, Gishen, Whitman, Gill, Barker and Walker (2016) found that Rounds helped to normalise emotional reactions and provided a useful space for reflection. At Plymouth University, we have attempted to run Schwartz round sessions with students. We have observed how these rounds seem to normalise emotions, aid the understanding of the roles of other professionals, and to encourage empathy with peers. Attendees have told us that speaking with other healthcare students has changed their perception of them in practice, meaning they feel more open and able to approach other healthcare students on the wards. Schwartz Rounds in the University context often provide healthcare students with one of their first exposures to students in other healthcare professions, allowing them to challenge stereotypes and see the human in the profession through discussions about the emotional impact of their work.

In practice, Universities have to consider a number of practical issues in running Rounds, such as voluntary or compulsory attendance, whether they form part of the curriculum, timing, locations and group size (Barker et al., 2016). At Plymouth University, there is a dedicated steering group of senior clinicians who are involved in teaching at the

University and are supported by the Point of Care Foundation. Trained facilitators and mentors support the recruitment of panellists and facilitation of Rounds. More information can be found on the Point of Care Foundation website about implementing Rounds (https://www.pointof-carefoundation.org.uk/our-work/schwartz-rounds/).

Schwartz Rounds are an example of where attempts at IPW have been translated into an interprofessional context (earlier in people's careers). However, most training efforts and interventions remain at the level of initial professional training, rather than later professional life. Schwarz rounds, in common with *Bridges*, enable contact between groups, but still do not explore the intricacies of working between professions in a pressurised work environment.

Training in Interprofessional Working for Professionals

The focus on interprofessional learning as students tackle challenges of IPW does not offer support to clinicians already in working practice. It treats clinicians as role models for students, yet some clinicians may struggle to model collaboration. It is already recognised that there can be very different ways of working in healthcare teams—interprofessional and multi-professional for example. The NHS suggests these are different, with multidisciplinary teams including people from different professions who maintain their own professional identities (Borrill et al., 2001; NHS England, 2014). In IPW, there can be a greater level of crossover, so that professionals might do very similar tasks—sometimes a speech therapist might do an assessment, sometimes a clinical psychologist. In these teams, clinicians were termed practitioners, rather than given a professional title.

Communication challenges from teamwork have also been identified. Recall Chapter 1, where we outlined the practice failures that occur through poor communication resulting in harm or discomfort to service users increased morbidity and mortality. Further, we also know that there are a number of issues for staff well-being, which is essential in maintaining values-based compassionate care (see Chapters 1 and 5). Addressing the challenges of IPW is not straightforward. As many researchers indicate (e.g. Weaver, Dy, & Rosen, 2014), understanding team working is complex, particularly given the dynamic nature of teams, meaning that how they operate differs in different organisations, at different times, and is dependent on the different ways in which teams are constituted. This book evidences this matter further. We have examined teams composing different numbers of staff, different levels of professional diversity, with different purposes, and achieving different clinical functions through different procedures. Furthermore, these teams all come from a particular region of the UK, so do not reflect the even more considerable, global diversity.

Some approaches to understanding IPW have focused on whole organisation designs. For example, in Canada, a number of organisational approaches have been implemented, where meeting space, and the environment, were changed in order to influence working practices (D'Amour, Goulet, Labadie, Martin-Rodriguez, & Pineault, 2008). This notion of environmental level change has been implemented in other areas, for example in the development of 'Psychological Environments' within some services (Johnson and Haigh, 2011). These broader interventions have shown some improvement in terms of addressing organisational cultures and provide a broader enabling approach to IPW. However, these interventions do not address the question of the things that people might actually say to each other in order to enable IPW. Other training packages available include online resources and information such as that provided by the Health Education Centres for North, Central, East and West London NHS (2012). These resources, which are openly accessible, considers the relevance to groups of themes such as stereotypes, social identity theory, learning theory and communities of practice. The approach provides different theoretical perspectives on multidisciplinary learning and encourages the reader to reflect on how some of these ideas might be relevant or beneficial to them. However, information for individuals alone is not enough, as IPW is inevitably a joint endeavour. Indeed, Lindqvist and Reeves (2007) emphasise that with clinicians in practice it can be useful to have regular meetings and debriefings in order to allow people opportunities to discuss the application of their training to practice. Thus, our training package was evolved both as something more formal than the Schwartz rounds and the Bridges projects already in place for students, to be more targeted, but also to maintain an emphasis on the importance of discussion and reflection, so that practitioners, as students could be engaged in their own learning and development.

The *MDTsInAction* Approach to Training Interprofessional Teams in Mental Health Services

In this section, we elaborate in more detail the approach that the *MDTsInAction* training took. Our training model draws on the following principles:

1. Insights learned from the interprofessional care literature, and the value-based approach of enhancing communication and compassion-focused care.
2. Insights developed from our *MDTsInAction* research project, based on an analysis of how clinicians interact within team meetings.
3. Insights drawn from our discursive psychology/conversation analysis approach to understanding interactions.
4. Insights from a clinical psychology/reflective practice approach to inform how to design the training.

Insights from Interprofessional Working and Our Research Programme

We attempted to take on board the now considerable evidence around the challenges faced by IPW. It seemed very relevant to make it clear that we were taking a values-based approach where we wanted to enhance communication to reduce poor outcomes, but also wanting to capture the range of different emotional and support issues that also seem crucial for staff well-being, and therefore ultimately, the delivery of care. Groups promoting IPW such as Schwarz rounds do operate within our local NHS services, but we wanted also to explore in the training programme how clinicians could make best use of the time that they had with each other, based on the findings from our research programme. For example, in the literature on interprofessional care, it is suggested that good communication and IPW can enhance emotional support. Aikman in Chapter 6 showed some interactional practices within team meetings that illustrate how this can be done. Parish in Chapter 8 showed how techniques such as repetition can ensure that issues are considered. In this way, we were in the unique position to offer examples of practices that were derived directly from observational evidence, and so illustrate some ways in which these outcomes could be achieved though interactional practices.

Insights from Discursive Psychology and Conversation Analysis

Through drawing on a discursive psychology/conversation analysis approach, we also suggest that we were able to address the 'theory-practice' gap. We had the advantage of having directly considered examples of actual practice in order to make sense of how to improve communication. Our method, conversation analysis, can have application in a number of ways (Antaki, 2011). Antaki suggested that this includes the identification of practices, which we have done here, and on other occasions extending from these to make recommendations. A further approach to applying Conversation Analysis has been introduced by Liz Stokoe (2014) as CARM. CARM shows how CA can become a training method which uses real-life recordings from conversations, rather than role-play. It has been shown to be hugely beneficial in offering training in mediation services. In this approach, workshop attendees are shown extracts from real-life mediation sessions. Part of the extract is played, and then participants are asked to anticipate what might come next. They then spend time thinking about the ways in which they were able to predict or not the next turn, and what this might mean for interactional outcomes. For example, this can be helpful in understanding how to obtain important information from people, particularly when they might be reluctant to offer it.

Insights from Clinical Psychology and Reflective Practice

In addition to these CA-based approaches, we also drew on the clinical psychology principle of reflective practice. CA is making moves into reflective practice contexts. For example, recent research has analysed what form of talk constitutes reflective practice (Veen & la Croix, 2017) and more relevantly, how the exploration of real-life events can promote reflexivity, based on the CARM method (Kirkwood, Jennings, Laurier, Cree, & Whyte, 2016).

We suggest that CA compliments approaches in reflective practice, by providing a way of looking at practice from the outside. Reflection can be described as a process of experiential learning where clinicians might (1) identify a particular action, (2) reflect on how it made them and others feel—what was helpful or not about it, (3) consider how to improve or change and then (4) repeat the cycle and monitor fresh feedback (Stedmon & Dallos, 2009). Schön (1983, 1987) similarly identified 'reflective practice' as a cyclical process which oscillates between thinking about past events and drawing on theoretical knowledge to connect with the experience of events in-the-moment. He draws a helpful distinction between a conscious process of looking back 'on-action' and a more spontaneous and intuitive process of reflecting 'in-action'. There are multiple structured models that draw on a reflective learning cycles (e.g. Gibbs, 1988; Johns, 1995) which have been applied across a range of professional training contexts (e.g. education, social work and nursing). We can also distinguish group and individual reflection. Group reflection seems to require additional components—a sense of group cohesion, trust and safety, and good facilitation (extracted from a literature review of Bailey and Graham, 2007; Dawber, 2013; Heneghan, Wright, & Watson, 2014; Knight, Sperlinger, & Maltby, 2010). Key features seem to include development of an emotional connection to the facilitator, clear boundaries, containment and validation of experiences, and the use of a questioning style encouraging reflective thinking. It is most often encouraged in the social context of supervision within mental health contexts.

These reflective approaches can be orientated to a particular theoretical approach which, to some extent will constrain the legitimate focus of the reflections themselves. For example, a psychoanalytic approach may focus on emotional contributions, a Cognitive Behavioural Therapy model may privilege consideration of how thoughts underpin actions, while a social constructionist perspective encourages exploration of multiple social influences on how meanings are constructed (Stedmon & Dallos, 2009). However, we also argue that these reflective approaches can be more focused in terms of developing and improving interprofessional relationships by focusing on conjoint team reflections around:

- **Relational actions**: that is how the team function together, relationships—professional and informal between team members, meanings and processes between people that occur.
- **Organisational actions**: that is the effects of the imposed structures of the organisation, such as how and where a meeting is conducted.
- **Clinical actions**: that is the clinical work accomplished in the meeting, such as allocating patients to particular services, representing service users, or producing a diagnosis.

These three areas of reflection were developed from a thematic analysis on the outputs from the *MDTsInAction* research programme. The programme developed from initial open questions around how MDTs function, and what may or may not constitute IPW. Through conversations with clinicians and service users over the 4 years of the project, we identified a range of key themes in terms of the direction of interest that service users, carers, clinicians and researchers were discussing in their research, which can be summarised by these three main themes. They therefore provided us with a framework for structuring the delivery of the training workshops, but also enabled us to be confident that these were recurrent themes in the areas of importance for training around interprofessional team working in multiple different mental health contexts. As the programme developed, these underpinned the framework that we used to organise and think about how each element of the research project might have an application.

Project Overview

Here, we outline the content and organisation of the training programme, and then we examine the ways that we have evaluated it. Our evaluation currently includes both questionnaires and feedback immediately post-sessions, and subsequent qualitative communications with teams and professionals collecting comments on the longer term effects of the training, and future recommendations.

Overview of the Training Programme

The main aims of the training programme were:

- To promote good relations between team members.
- To promote awareness for members of the team of how the team works together.
- To increase understanding of how language works in teams.
- Understanding how to develop IPW/interdisciplinary working.

Our training sessions were 1.5 hours each, and we ran 4 sessions with different teams and groups of individuals. The training developed over a 3-year period. The initial two training sessions were held as part of CPD events and were more generic in their nature in terms of focusing on specific interactional features such as adjacency pairs, e.g. question and answer sequences, that were relatively straightforward to identify. The later sessions were much more specific.

In the final version, sessions were based around an introduction to team function, clinical practices and organisational issues. We began with an introduction to IPW, and then we discussed examples and read examples of each type of interaction to illustrate some of the different effects that occur in language as we speak, taken from the research presented within this book. We then provided practitioners the time and space to discuss and reflect on how these events were relevant to their own practice.

We defined relational activities as including: emotional support; professional identities and relationships and power relationships. We focused on one area within these and provided a related short transcript which people listened to, and we then discussed it in terms of relational activities in teams. Although we had a range of examples, we found that in a 1.5 hours session, only one of each type of activity (relational, organisational or clinical) was enough. As an example, we include here Extract 1 which was used to discuss findings around relational activities.

Extract 1: Institutional Agenda Change Through Professional Validation

```
1    Bob:        →      I I'm sure Richard will make sure it:'s

2                →      >discussed< with all doctors

3    Sandra:            fab that's ↓great >okay< fifte:en PIM:S↑

4                       Sue's gonna ↑y:eah↓ a

5                       [ring I still  think that's

6    Sue:               [I a:m ↓yea
```

Extract 1 was selected as it illustrates how we can challenge the suggestion that a claim to be a doctor is necessarily a claim to have power 'over'

others in the meeting (see Chapter 5). Instead, here Bob uses his professional status to enhance his claim of assurance that 'all' doctors will be
informed. We found it useful to use this short extract to help to reflect
on the different ways that phrases could be interpreted, and the assumptions which are used to interpret the meaning of utterances. Within some
groups, for example, there were tensions in terms of knowledge from
different professions—the 'meaning' of people's statements was assumed
based on knowledge of their profession or role. However, by taking apart
this small extract and analysing talk at a turn by turn level, these tensions were removed so that clinicians could think about what a statement
did in an interaction, and were both less likely to apply evaluative judge-
ments and more likely to be aware when they were making them.

The second main theme of the workshops emergent from the
MDTsInAction Research programme was organisational activities. We
defined these as related to meeting structure, such as the use of an
agenda or not, meeting roles, and record keeping. In order to stimu-
late discussion here about the organisation of meetings, we played two
extracts. Firstly, Extract 2, illustrating how the agenda is used by team
members.

Extract 2: Using the Agenda

```
1   Sue:      °rather than developing several reports.°

2   Sandra:   Yeap. uhm.

3             I know >it is on the< agenda but it's

4             just the kind

5             of the the focus of that °slightly°↓

6   Sandra:   and do we know generally what

7             the feedback was?

8   Sue:      >We can pick it up on the< ↑agend:a
```

Secondly, we included Extract 3, to help to illustrate the ways that the agenda was important.

Extract 3: No Agenda

```
1   GRA:      °ri:ght°, okay .hhh >I haven't

2             actually got an< agenda

3             s:o ↑umm(.)

4             hu-hu-hu Milly was organising it, Jenny

5             was supposed to chair a:nnnnnnnd↑ hhh.

6             she's not `er:e↑ (.)

7   KAT:      [>So what [would be usefu-<

8   AMY:      [Okay so what

9   GRA:      [She's got GOT po:::orly po::rly

10            children [unfortunately

11  KAT:        [So what'd be usefu:l to do in

12            this meeting >do you< °think°

13  GRA:      Errr actually I'm going to thr:ow it

14            back to Maddie because um she's↑su.hh knows

15            what she wants to cover ↓within thi:s

16  MAD:      Right. One of th:e initial things wa:s that

17            Jilly wa::s >consulting the background<

18            Jilly was really (.) em poorly↓

19            mentally .hh unmwell.
```

The use of these two extracts enabled practitioners to reflect together on the ways that the very organisation of conversations in meetings affects how interactions occur. With the agenda, talk can be more ordered— turn-taking is easier, and people are able to use the agenda to present the points that they want to, by referring to the agenda (Extract 2). However, when people are very used to working in a particular way, meetings can be less successful without this structure (no agenda, as in Extract 3). Extract 3 usefully illustrates how attempts at removing meeting hierarchy can work, and led to discussions of how to most effectively use meeting spaces, and what purposes this can serve.

Finally, we considered clinical activities, under which we included advocacy, advice giving, decision-making and clinical formulations. For this section we used an example of a checking question, as in Extract 4, to illustrate that it is possible to prioritise service delivery over organisational activities:

Extract 4: Prioritising Services Over Meeting Organisation

```
1   Jane:      okay lovely right MRI

2              scans procedures

3              right we we can take that off now

4   Zoe:       is that sorted

5   Jane:      I think Richard was going to go

6              do you know anything
```

The last extract was useful, but for future sessions, we suggest that it might be more helpful to reflect and discuss other features, such as repetition in order to open up the floor for discussion where an implied decision is being queried as in Chapter 8, or to examine formulations as in Chapter 7.

Recommendations for Interprofessional Team Working

- Staff appreciate continued training around communications within their team, and methods of improving team working practices. We therefore suggest that it is appropriate for all teams to continue to engage with this form of development.
- Staff suggested that this opportunity enabled people to help to think about how to include delicate issues or concerns within their team meetings, and therefore regular training might be beneficial for staff to identify where their practice is more or less beneficial.
- Staff teams benefit from bringing in people to facilitate discussions of their team meeting practice, in terms of reflecting on organisational, team and clinical activities conducted, and how these can he enhanced.
- Staff teams benefit from recording and discussing their own conversations, once initial training has been offered in the basic principles of conversation analysis and encouraging participants to regard language as functional.

Summary

There are a wide range of IPE initiatives currently being developed across the globe. These include didactic teaching during training programmes and also the evolution of more creative approaches such as Schwartz rounds and student-led interdisciplinary initiatives. With the exception of Schwartz rounds, most of these interventions have focused on IPE for those still in training, rather than supporting clinicians already in post. Some IPW interventions have included the restructuring or re-organisation of environments, but few have focused more directly on how to interact in meetings. Training around meetings talk, using direct examples of interactions was an effective way of making training relevant to clinical work. It ensured that the situations considered were exactly like those that practitioners might encounter. Clinicians enthusiastically attended the training sessions and commented on the advantages of not only being offered practical learning, but also updated skills around how different forms of qualitative research can be relevant to their work. Some clinicians had little understanding of the research technique and enjoyed this approach. They also commented that they were able to see how this was relevant to enhancing ability to reflect on team practices. Learning occurred not only around the strategies that other teams used (as reported), but also enhancing the awareness of clinicians of how they were interacting with each other, so that they had more skills to think about the ways in which their communication might affect those of others. Future research would need to develop the training further.

References

Antaki, C. (Ed.). (2011). Applied conversation analysis: Intervention and change in institutional talk. Basingstoke: Palgrave Macmillan.

Bailey, M. E., & Graham, M. G. (2007). Introducing guided group reflective practice in an Irish palliative care unit. *International Journal of Palliative Nursing, 13*(11), 555–560.

Barker, R., Cornwell, J., & Gishen, F. (2016). Introducing compassion into the education of health care professionals; can Schwartz Rounds help? *Journal of Compassionate Health Care, 3*(3). https://doi.org/10.1186/s40639-016-0020-0.

Boet, S., Bould, M. D., Burn, L., & Reeves, S. (2014). Twelve tips for a successful interprofessional team-based high-fidelity simulation education session. *Medical Teacher, 36*(10), 853–857. https://doi.org/10.3109/0142159x.2014.923558.

Borrill, C. S., Carletta, J., Carter, A. J., Dawson, J. F., Garrod, S. Rees, A., …, West, M. A. (2001). *The effectiveness of health care teams in the National Health Service*. Aston University. Retrieved on 10 May 2016 from http://homepages.inf.ed.ac.uk/jeanc/DOH-final-report.pdf.

D'Amour, D., Goulet, L., Labadie, J., Martin-Rodriguez, L. S., & Pineault, R. (2008). A model and typology of collaboration between professionals in healthcare organisations. *BMC Health Services Research, 8*, 188. https://doi.org/10.1186/1472-6963-8-188.

Dawber, C. (2013). Reflective practice groups for nurses: A consultation liaison psychiatry nursing initiative: Part 2—The evaluation. *International Journal of Mental Health Nursing, 22,* 241–248.

Francis, R. (2010). *Independent inquiry into care provided by Mid Staffordshire NHS Foundation Trust.* London: The Stationary Office.

Francis, R. (2013). *Report of the Mid Staffordshire NHS Foundation Trust Public Inquiry Volume 1: Analysis of evidence and lessons learned (Part 1).* London: The Stationary Office.

George, M. (2016). Stress in NHS staff triggers defensive inward-focussing and an associated loss of connection with colleagues: This is reversed by Schwartz Rounds. *Journal of Compassionate Health Care, 3*(9). https://doi.org/10.1186/s40639-016-0025-8.

Gibbs, G. (1988). *Learning by doing: A guide to teaching and learning methods.* Oxford: Oxford Further Education Unit.

Gishen, F., Whitman, S., Gill, D., Barker, R., & Walker, S. (2016). Schwartz Centre Rounds: A new initiative in the undergraduate curriculum—What do medical students think? *BMC Medical Education, 16.* https://doi.org/10.1186/s12909-016-0762-6.

General Medical Council (GMC). (2015). *Promoting excellence: Standards for medical education and training.* Retrieved 2 January 2018 from http://www.gmc-uk.org/education/standards.asp.

Goodrich, J. (2011). *Schwartz center rounds: Evaluation of the UK pilots.* London: The Kings Fund.

Health Education Centres for North, Central, East and West London NHS. (2012). *Multiprofessional faculty development: Interprofessional Education.* Retrieved on 21 June 2018 from https://faculty.londondeanery.ac.uk/e-learning/interprofessional-education.

Heneghan, C., Wright, J., & Watson, G. (2014). Clinical psychologists' experiences of reflective staff groups in inpatient psychiatric settings: A mixed methods study. *Clinical Psychology and Psychotherapy, 21,* 324–340.

Hooper, C., Meakin, R., & Jones, M. (2005). Where do students go when they are ill: How medical students access health care. *Medical Education, 39*(6), 588–593. https://doi.org/10.1111/j.1365-2929.2005.02175.x.

Johns, C. (1995). Framing learning through reflection within Carper's fundamental ways of knowing in nursing. *Journal of Advanced Nursing, 22*(2), 226–234.

Johnson, R., & Haigh, R. (2011). Social psychiatry and social policy for the 21st century: New concepts for new needs—The 'enabling Environments' initiative. *Mental Health and Social Inclusion, 15*(1), 17–23.

Kirkwood, S., Jennings, B., Laurier, E., Cree, A., & Whyte, B. (2016). Towards an interactional approach to reflective practice in social work. *European Journal of Social Work, 19*(3–4), 484–499.

Knight, K., Sperlinger, D., & Maltby, M. (2010). Exploring the personal and professional impact of reflective practice groups: A survey of 18 cohorts from a UK clinical psychology training course. *Clinical Psychology and Psychotherapy, 17,* 427–437.

Lindqvist, S. M., & Reeves, S. (2007). Facilitators' perceptions of delivering interprofessional education: A qualitative study. *Medical Teacher, 29*(4), 403–405. https://doi.org/10.1080/01421590701509662.

Maben, J., Taylor, C., Dawson, J., Leamy, M., McCarthy, I., Reynolds, E., …, Foot, C. (2017). *A realist informed mixed methods evaluation of Schwartz Center Rounds in England.* Accessed 2 January 2018 from https://njl-admin.nihr.ac.uk/document/download/2011408.

NHS England. (2014). *MDT development: Working towards an effective multi-disciplinary team.* NHS England: Leeds.

Nursing and Midwifery Council (NMC). (2010). *Standards for pre-registration nursing education.* Retrieved 2 January 2018 from https://www.nmc.org.uk/globalassets/sitedocuments/standards/nmc-standards-for-pre-registration-nursing-education.pdf.

Pecukonis, E., Doyle, O., & Bliss, D. L. (2008). Reducing barriers to interprofessional training: Promoting interprofessional cultural competence. *Journal of Interprofessional Care, 22*(4), 417–428. https://doi.org/10.1080/13561820802190442.

Point of Care Foundation. (2015). *Schwartz Rounds.* Retrieved from http://www.pointofcarefoundation.org.uk/our-work/Schwartz-rounds/.

Reed, E., Cullen, A., Gannon, C., Knight, A., & Todd, J. (2015). Use of Schwartz Centre Rounds in a UK hospice: Findings from a longitudinal evaluation. *Journal of Interprofessional Care, 29*(4), 365–366. https://doi.org/10.3109/13561820.2014.983594.

Robert, G., Philippou, J., Leamy, M., Reynolds, E., Ross, S., Bennett, L., …, Maben, J. (2017). Exploring the adoption of Schwartz Center Rounds as an organisational innovation to improve staff well-being in England, 2009–2015. *BMJ Open, 7.* https://doi.org/10.1136/bmjopen-2016-014326.

Roberts, L., Warner, T., & Trumpower, D. (2000). Medical students' evolving perspectives on their personal health care: Clinical and educational implications of a longitudinal study. *Comprehensive Psychiatry, 41*(4), 303–314. https://doi.org/10.1053/comp.2000.0410303.

Schön, D. A. (1983). *The reflective practitioner: How professionals think in action*. New York: Basic Books.

Schön, D. A. (1987). *Educating the reflective practitioner: Toward a new design for teaching and learning in the professions*. San Francisco, CA: Jossey-Bass.

Schwartz, B. (1995). *A patient's story*. Retrieved from http://www.theschwartz-center.org/media/patient_story.pdf.

Stedmon, J., & Dallos, R. (2009). *Reflective practice in psychotherapy and counselling*. Maidenhead: Open University Press.

Stokoe, E. (2014). The Conversation Analytic Role-play Method (CARM): A Method for training communication skills as an alternative to simulated role-play. *Research on Language and Social Interaction, 47*(3), 255–265. https://doi.org/10.1080/08351813.2014.925663.

Weaver, S. J., Dy, S. M., & Rosen, M. A. (2014). Team-training in healthcare: A narrative synthesis of the literature. *BMJ Quality and Safety, 23*, 359–372. https://doi.org/10.1136/bmjqs-2013-001848.

Veen, M., & la Croix, A. (2017). The swamplands of reflection: Using conversation analysis to reveal the architecture of group reflection sessions. *Medical Education, 51*(3), 324–336.

16

Conclusions: Advancing Team Working in Community Mental Health Settings

Cordet Smart and Timothy Auburn

Introduction

This book has sought to develop an understanding of collaborative team working through the methodological lenses of conversation analysis and discursive psychology. The chapters in this book have focused on team meeting contexts, where it was possible to record and analyse in detail how clinicians directly communicate with each other. As we stated in Chapter 1, the project began with discussions in the course of our everyday work, reflecting on practice during the training of clinical psychologists. From just a few brief conversations, it has blossomed into a substantive raft of work that still has only really touched the surface of how we might better understand how staff discursively accomplish

C. Smart (✉) · T. Auburn
School of Psychology, University of Plymouth, Plymouth, UK
e-mail: cordet.smart@plymouth.ac.uk

T. Auburn
e-mail: T.Auburn@plymouth.ac.uk

© The Author(s) 2018
C. Smart and T. Auburn (eds.), *Interprofessional Care and Mental Health*,
The Language of Mental Health, https://doi.org/10.1007/978-3-319-98228-1_16

collaboration with each other. An important aim of this work has been to develop future training programmes to match practitioners' needs.

This programme of work was new and bold at its outset—there was little extant discursive or conversation analytic research which explored the functioning of MDTs. We received some resistance to our methodological approach. Clinicians endorsed the need for this research, but academics and ethics boards struggled to distinguish the potential insights of conversation analysis from other less intensive forms of research on communication. They argued that there are already 'principles' of communication that are known—such as developing trust, or the importance of psychological safety in teams. However, those who have then re-read our work have begun to see that what a detailed examination of talk adds is an understanding of how these phenomenological experiences may be constituted within the interactions that staff have on a daily basis. Clinicians in particular have commented on how difficult it is to translate the principles of practice outlined in health policies into systematic ways of working. Our approach, however, has been able to produce findings that are directly relevant to individual clinicians' practice.

We hope, then, that this work provides the foundations for new understandings of team processes, and how relational, organisational and clinical activities are conducted in the daily work of clinicians working in mental health settings (and beyond). In this concluding chapter we will provide an overview of the main findings of the chapters and draw out the principle themes that can contribute to interprofessional working in mental health contexts.

Overview

The book has taken us on a rapid tour of the *MDTsInAction* research project. Chapter 1 set out the rationale for developing a better understanding of communication between professionals who provide mental health, and related, services. The principle communication problems evident in health care working were identified. These problems are wide ranging not least because of the multiple modes of communication (e.g. face to face, telephone, email and report writing). The review summarised the frequently dramatic effects for service users of poor communication across health care—from cancelled operations to the wrong intervention. Hospital stays are often increased where communication is poor, and the service user's perspective is frequently overlooked or misinterpreted. Organisational outcomes included increased time on each case and resource saturation, and staff effects included those on reputation and job satisfaction, sometimes leading to burnout. How 'power' is enfolded into the organisational hierarchy was also identified as contributing to communication difficulties. One of the greatest sources of difficulties was where there was limited opportunity for, and poor quality of, face-to-face communications. It was based on issues like these that we developed the *MDTsInAction* research programme. It aimed to explore how the emergent use of team-based approaches to patient care worked on practice and in particular in team meeting contexts.

Part I (Chapters 2 and 3) then considered methodological issues. In Chapter 2, we set out our main approach based on conversation analysis and discursive psychology as a framework for understanding the interactional processes underlying multidisciplinary team meetings. The chapter advocated conversation analysis/discursive psychology as an essential approach for understanding the nature of the interaction that takes place between professionals in meetings. The key principles of conversation analysis were briefly summarised, namely turn taking, sequence organisation and repair. Discursive psychology was described as building upon conversation analysis but with a particular focus on the discursive deployment of psychological terminology. This approach was illustrated by taking the issue of 'trust' as this concept has often been invoked as a necessary precondition to effective team working. Discursive psychology encourages us to explore how notions like trust are constituted in talk as forms of action and how they are oriented to managing participants' concerns.

Chapter 3 examined the ethical concerns which attended the project. It sought to bring together concerns raised by the unique context of the research, that is, integrating the study of mental health care contexts, with the value of service user involvement and engagement, particularly as service users were often absent from the multidisciplinary meetings themselves. We also considered how this fitted with conversation analysis as a methodology and the implications for researchers, clinicians, service users and consultants. One overriding issue concerned the extent of participation and involvement of the different stakeholders (health care professionals, service users). In the *MDTsInAction* project, we sought to engage our stakeholders fully in all stages of the project. This approach facilitated our working relationships and also enabled learning to flow more easily between researchers and other stakeholders involved (health care professionals, service user consultants, service manager consultants). Thus, we attempted to use insights from our literature review in Chapter 1, around the challenges of power and hierarchy, to inform the ethical design of the *MDTsInAction* research project, as well as to later focus the analysis on relevant topics.

Part II focused on some of the broader institutional features of MDT meetings, such as how they were located in particular contexts, how power was a central issue, and how staff relationships seemed to work within these contexts.

Chapter 4 outlined the unique way in which conversation analysis conceptualises context. Context is regarded as endogenously constituted by the participants themselves rather than imposed upon participants from above by the institution. This way of understanding context in turn suggested that we should look at the meeting talk itself for evidence of how participants oriented to and displayed collaborative working. We argued that such collaboration was displayed in the 'mundane' interactions which themselves constituted the meetings as MDT meetings. By using some brief extracts from MDT meetings, we demonstrated both how meeting members in a mundane sense collaboratively achieved the work of the meeting and displayed their organisational and work-related concerns in their turns of talk.

Within MDTs, there are often multiple and varied contexts to which participants orientate, and through our substantive consultation and literature reviews, we identified the relevance of four main contexts—interpersonal, interprofessional, local service context and national policy context related to service delivery. We then illustrated how very subtle checking questions or use of different terms can be used to orientate to these various contexts—'we' in terms of membership of the local team; checking questions to consider local service provision, and how the chair was treated as in charge of the meeting.

This chapter was important as in our discussions with clinicians on training for joined up working, they had argued that much of this training had not addressed the particulars of their working context. So, for example, it is fine to suggest that teams need more time for face-to-face communication, or that they need to problem-solve in a particular way, but being able to draw clinicians' attention to the practical ways in which they conduct team meetings was much more helpful for them in thinking how to implement these sorts of recommendations.

Teams also differed in the sorts of remit they were following. For example, for one of our expert-by-experience consultants, it was surprising that the psychiatrist was not the lead figure in community learning disability teams. However, in these teams the main work was often concerned with providing ongoing support to ensure that people with learning disabilities are successful in their everyday lives, and so social workers, nurses or psychologists sometimes had more knowledge of support in this area. Teams also commented on how the national contexts affected their working practices—when there was national critique of social care, this was felt in their work. The location of teams within their context for any subsequent training, and to understand the meaning of the ideas and practices, is therefore key—both to ensure that training and research that is developed is relevant to clinical practice, and to enable clinicians to be able to relate to how this is relevant and so apply it.

Chapter 5 followed on with an analysis of how power worked in MDTs. Power, as set out in Chapter 1, was central to the book. In this chapter, Heritage's work on epistemics, and in particular epistemic authority was set out alongside a consideration of deontic authority. These types of authority can be considered as ways of assserting power or influence. We saw in this chapter how the service user's needs could be prioritised in such a way that those with relevant knowledge were accorded greater influence on the basis of their epistemic status and stance. We also saw here how their historical, as well as personal knowledge of the service user was valued in learning disability contexts, over and above that of the professional knowledge of other speakers such as the psychiatrist. These historical perspectives are more significant in community learning disability settings than say acute mental health where service users may be less known to staff. This is another example of where the context of the setting was important for understanding how other features of team interaction work. A further theme that developed from this chapter on power was the way in which the team was able to operate as a group to provide space for others to speak, or to close down particular speakers.

Chapter 6 explored what Aikman termed the 'unintended' consequences of team interactions. This chapter directly linked to some of the key concerns seen with poor communication in practice, namely staff burnout and the delivery of compassionate care. She suggests that team members often seek help, air frustrations and name tensions within the team, and that these different practices can be used to support staff and to create spaces of psychological safety. These practices also connect with staff well-being and therefore the staff's continued ability to deliver compassionate care. This chapter illustrates also how some of the broader guidelines for interprofessional practice might be practically implemented through recognisable interactional practices. Clinicians can benefit from reflecting on discourse as providing a range of options for talking about team concerns and that some options are more likely to create supportive team contexts.

Part III focused on the clinical activities of meetings, such as formulations. Formulation (Chapter 7) is a central concept in Clinical Psychology and indeed within mental health care more broadly. Psychological formulation involves examining the broader social and psychological circumstances for the individual, to reveal cycles that maintain behaviours that are socially challenging. Peckitt showed that team formulation is enhanced by the multiple insights that different practitioners can provide. However, despite team formulation being frequently theorised and discussed, it was difficult to identify these events in team interactions. Team formulations were noticeably unmarked; they were often introduced tentatively and enabled delicate and emotional views to be presented alongside the formulation itself.

Chapter 8 examined MDT meetings which were concerned with whether or not to assign children a diagnosis of autism. The chapter explored the different ways in which information was delivered which led to more open team discussions of the child's circumstances. Parish identified three significant practices: presenting information with marked uncertainty, making interjections and using repetition to make a previous contribution 'noteworthy'. These practices are particularly relevant for reflecting on how increased involvement can be gained within team meetings. They differed from some of the chapters which had identified extended multi-unit turns, for example storytelling, as practices for introducing complex patient information.

Chapter 9 focused on how clinicians might elicit help from each other within MDTs, particularly when services are overstretched. The chapter illustrates how a 'stepwise transition' can be observed where people move from the discourse marker 'maybe' then using the modal verb 'might' and the pro-term 'somebody'. The chair's role within this process was again noted in this chapter—as the main person to take up the response. Chairs often resisted the request for help particularly in the terms proposed by the requester. It was notable here that to support interprofessional working greater egalitarianism was needed so that the chair could consider allowing other team members to respond to requests directly.

Chapter 10 described how diagnostic meetings worked within a memory clinic. One main finding was that there were considerable differences in the ways in which the assessors of the person living with demential (PLD) and of their supporter presented their information. Descriptions of interactions between the service user and their assessor were included only by the service user assessor. The assessor of the supporter directly reported the supporter's interactions with the service user. Furthermore, the assessors often spoke as if they were part of the family themselves. Dickenson makes the point that this practice diminishes the voice of the person living with dementia themselves. Previous research suggested that people with memory difficulties often report the experience of not being heard or listened to. In this setting, there was a risk that this experience could be amplified. However, this raised the question of what other approaches would be acceptable to represent information about the service user's thoughts and feelings. This chapter provides a sobering account of how a person's memory difficulties are discursively constructed and the potential consequences for the person's identity.

Part IV focused on patient-centred interactions and how service users are represented within multidisciplinary meetings. The first chapter (Chapter 11) in this section examined how service users can be advocated for within MDTs. In certain situations, service users might either be at risk of not being offered services for their needs, or might be identified as not receiving appropriate services. When this occurs, a team member will present an extended telling of a story that accounts for why people should have access to services. Smart and Reed showed how key devices were used within these tellings to persuade the team to provide services—for example a personal emotional statement from a clinician 'It worries me', use of reported speech (direct or indirect), re-enactment of a difficult situation or the use of contrast structures between different opinions about the service user's needs.

Chapter 12 examined occasions where clinicians raised concerns about service users. Tremblett identified five practices using the word concern: firstly, as openers whereby this term seems to open up discussion. Secondly, concerns can be owned by a speaker, rather than shared, which allows the speaker to engage in an extended turn. If they are initiated earlier, these concern constructions are more complex in so far as they require more accounting than if they follow on from a wider discussion. Where the concern has been raised by someone not present, there is a greater degree of evaluation of the concern. Alternatively, where there is 'no concern' then conversations are immediately shut down. In all reported cases, these concerns were related to risk, which in part accounts for the way in which they work to open up discussions. Awareness of these diverse practices for introducing 'concerns' can be helpful for clinicians in promoting interprofessional communication.

Whiter, Durkin and Tauchert (Chapter 13) brought more fully into view the perspective of the service user. Whiter analysed with two people who were living with psychosis, a focus group discussion of clinicians who worked as members of an early intervention in psychosis team. This chapter was included to provide a different perspective on how we understand what might be lost in some staff interactions. Whiter identified within the clinicians' discourse four linguistic repertoires through which they understood and constructed psychosis. These repertoires are interesting in themselves, but to take this analysis further, Whiter recorded her own and her colleagues' response to these repertoires. This second level analysis suggested that the development of a shared language between service users and staff is important. This serves as a reminder that where we have sought to examine conversations and this can seem removed from clinical practice to clinicians, it might seem even more removed from reality for service users. Further, the chapter illustrated how good intentions such as moving to words such as 'experience' or 'insight' can sometimes too easily become translated back into less psycho-social and more diagnostic or categorical ways of understanding mental health. Importantly, the reflections show how service users can bring a unique and valuable perspective to the research process.

Part V focused on some of the interventions that we developed based on the project. This included firstly our use of joint analysis, presented in Chapter 14. Here, we reported the way that we engaged not only in data groups with other conversation analysts to discuss data, but also how we designed sessions to engage our participants and support the research process. For example, we presented extracts where we (the researchers) had the greatest uncertainty, or where we wanted to check our analysis or the transcription process. This enabled us to check the relevance of our work to clinicians themselves, as it was their practice that we sought to develop.

Finally, in Chapter 15 we tried to bring together some of the main thinking within the book and to show how we had transformed this into a training approach. We situated our training workshops as drawing on work from approaches to interprofessional education (IPE), reflective practice and conversation analysis. We summarised our overall model as having developed into three different domains of activities that we see as happening within MDTs—relational activities (such as the negotiation of personal and professional relationships); organisational activities (such as the negotiation of the agenda and service priorities); and clinical activities (such as advocating and formulating for service users).

Summary: Main Themes

Throughout the book, there have been a number of recurrent themes. In this last section, we take the opportunity to summarise these principle themes.

Representing Service User Needs in MDT Meetings

Representation of service user needs was one of the main tasks of professionals within MDT meetings, whether this is for individual service users as in diagnostic or allocations meetings, or for client groups, as in manager or business meetings. This task took on a particular importance as more often than not, the service user was absent from the meeting itself. As discussed in Chapter 3, the main resistance to our project from funding and ethics boards was around why it is relevant to invest money and time on a project that does not directly engage with service users as participants. The answer, of course, is that many decisions are made where service users are not present. There are multiple reasons for this absence: to avoid service user burden; logistical imperatives for the rapid review of multiple service users; and of assembling clinicians together in one place.

Representation of service users was achieved in a number of ways. Chapter 11 specifically examined how clinicians were able to advocate for service users, but each chapter in the book illustrates ways in which service users' needs and concerns were discussed. We were able to identify illustrations of compassion in how staff can be supported to help service users in Chapter 6, to key practices for opening discussions. Most insightful, however, was to hear the reflections of service users themselves (see Chapter 13), as well as from our project consultants. The book draws attention to how the representation of service users within these meetings is constrained by the format and context of the meetings, the purpose of the meetings, who is present, and how well they know the service users.

Engaging Clinicians with Different Professional Backgrounds and Experience

The second main theme concerned how to enhance participation of those from different professional backgrounds and in different positions within the hierarchical structure of health and social care services. Throughout the book, a number of practices have been identified that can facilitate engagement, such as using the term 'concern', or querying an assessment. Other forms of gaining credibility include the use of direct reported speech, or historical claims about the experience of the service user. We were also able to evidence how 'relevance to the service user under discussion' can be more important in these community teams, as a gateway to participation, than medical training. It is suggested that this foci as a stated aim of team meetings might help more staff to feel open in participating within team meetings. Thus, despite the evidence of hierarchies as problematic, we were able to show good practice, where relevance to the service user and compassionate care was often prioritised.

Service User Involvement and Participation in CA/DP Research on MDT Meetings

This book dealt in multiple places with the challenges of involving people at different levels. The project itself included within the team people with lived experience of mental distress and also consulted with multiple stakeholder groups. This involvement was essential, particularly as our focus was on meetings where service users were absent, and arguably this form of involvement might therefore stand to offer some governance to these occasions. Involvement was also included when we implemented joint analysis. We do suggest that analysis with stakeholders is undertaken separately to research focused data groups, as it might be confusing and alienating to mix the two, unless the service user or clinician has a desire to learn conversation analysis. However, the additional consideration of context and experience from those whose lives are affected by these events, we hope, lends greater compassion and answers the concerns of any who might consider CA as a more academic exercise. The involvement of stakeholders in this way seems congruent with a concern for naturalistic relevance of the findings.

Learning Points for Researchers in the Field

This book set out not only to report our findings for how a CA/DP approach has provided insight into practices in MDT meetings, but also to provide some learning points for future researchers. Significant challenges were identified in our work through the combination of our topic, the context of mental health care research and the use of CA as a method. Some chapters have included reflective learning points and overall we have attempted to move back and forward between academic insights from CA and DP, to experiences in the real-life world of MDTs in various mental health settings. To summarise, we suggest some key learning points:

- If you can, be part of a team of researchers (which could be a supervisory team for a postgraduate student) and network to include service users, carers, knowledgable conversation analysts or discursive psychologists, clinicians and specialists in the area that you are working with—this helps the researchers to reflect some of the diversity of interpretations and gives greater opportunity for developing credibility of the work.
- Try to liaise with different disciplines and access networks that cross professional boundaries. This is sometimes easier or harder, depending on the discipline, but it is helpful to think about the learning from the research that we are conducting and apply it to how the research team itself works. Try to be open and consider issues that might cross boundaries. For example, working in the best interests of the service user.
- Organise and attend regular data groups, and when planning for joint analysis, groups remember to plan enough time to prepare the data first.
- In discussions with others, try not to be dissuaded. Being open and honest in explaining the research and the rationale and taking on board the applied concerns is valuable. Indeed, for a successful project, the CA analyst might have to spend considerable time consulting with service users, and other stakeholders, to capture the priorities for knowledge for specific MDT contexts.

The book is also an illustration that students at all levels can engage with these projects—work is presented from undergraduate, masters, Ph.D. and clinical doctorate students, all of whom were able to contribute. We would suggest that the main secret to this is to keep projects as targeted as possible and not to be concerned about exploring one phenomenon in detail and overlooking other things. Ultimately, as described in Chapter 4, we can see the broader context within the details of the interaction, and although early in the analysis it might be hard to see where things are going, perseverance wins through.

Appendix: Jeffersonian Transcription Conventions

For a fuller discussion of these transcription conventions, see Hepburn, H., & Bolden, G. (2013). The conversation analytic approach to transcription. In J. Sidnell & T. Stivers (Eds.), *Handbook of conversation analysis*. Chichester: Wiley-Blackwell.

[text] [text]	Square brackets indicated the start and finish of overlapping talk
=	Equals sign indicates latching where there is no discernible gap between the end of one turn and the start of the next
	Equals signs can also show a speaker's talk broken up into separate lines on the transcript to accommodate the placement of overlapping talk
(number)	Silences in talk (gaps or pauses) are indicated by a number in brackets. Silences are normally timed to the nearest tenth of a second
.	A full stop indicates a falling intonation often characteristic of the end of a turn

C. Smart and T. Auburn (eds.), *Interprofessional Care and Mental Health*, The Language of Mental Health, https://doi.org/10.1007/978-3-319-98228-1

?	A question mark indicates a strongly rising (questioning) intonation though it does not necessarily indicate that the phrase is a question
,	A comma indicates a more weakly rising intonation
<u>Text</u>	Underlining indicates emphasis placed on the underlined word or part of word
↓ or ↑	Down and up arrows indicated more marked lowering or raising of pitch
>text< or <text>	Greater than and less than symbols indicate a speeding up or slowing down of the talk contained between the symbols
<	A less than symbol on its own indicates that the following talk is 'left pushed' into the previous talk
:	Colons are used to indicate stretching of a sound in a word. The number of colons is proportional to the length of the 'stretch'
-	A hyphen at the end of work or part of a word indicates that the word was cut off
£text£	Pound signs indicate that the text enclosed by them is said in a 'smiley' voice
#text#	Hash sign indicates that the talk enclosed by the sign is said in a 'creaky' voice
hhh .hhh	Aspiration is indicated by 'h', the number of h's is proportional to the length of the aspiration. A series of h's indicates out-breath. A series of h's preceded by a full stop indicates in-breath
hah/huh etc. wo(h)rd	Sounds of laughter are shown as separate laughter particles Bracketed h shows laughter particles contained in words
((text))	Text contained within double brackets indicates the transcriber's comments

Glossary

Adjacency pair Is a two-part exchange in which the second utterance is functionally dependent on the first, as exhibited in conventional greetings, invitations and requests. The first utterance is called the first pair part (FPP) or the first turn. The second or responding utterance is called the second pair part (SPP) or the second turn

Affiliation According with the demonstrated emotional stance of the speaker of a prior turn

Alignment According with the expected next sequential turn, for example, following a question with an answer

Autism Spectrum Disorder ASD is a neurodevelopmental condition which is lifelong and causes impairments in communication, rigidity of thinking and cognitive ability

Bakhtian Discourse analysis This is an approach to analysing discourse that is grounded in the work of Bakhtin, which conceptualises language as dialogue and a site of ongoing struggle

Collocate To utter a word or phrase alongside or in close proximity to another in a 'frozen' or semi-formulaic way

Co-morbid When there is more than one co-existing health condition or diagnoses

C. Smart and T. Auburn (eds.), *Interprofessional Care and Mental Health*, The Language of Mental Health, https://doi.org/10.1007/978-3-319-98228-1

Concrete competence Problem-solving strategies that are based on lived or concrete experiences

Critical Discourse Analysis An umbrella term that refers to a collection of discourse analytic perspectives that emerged in the early 1990s, which attends generally to criticality, power and ideology, among other constructs. It often attends to the way in which power is produced in and through discourses and structures

Critical Discursive Psychology This is an approach to analysing discourse that considers both the individual's psychological representation in how they talk and how they are politically positioned

Deconstructionism Typically associated with the work of Derrida, it is a theoretical position that challenges the assumptions generally held about certainty and truth arguing that words only can refer to other words, and thus attempts to show how statements about text subvert their own meaning

Discursive Psychology A discourse analytic approach developed by Edwards and Potter (1992) which focused on the psychological language people use to describe mental states to perform a social action. This is a form of analysis of the details of interaction and how these are related to psychological concepts and ideas such as emotions and thoughts

Discursive Repertoires Are frequently used phrases or explanations that a speaker might use to explain something (see Linguistic Repertoires)

Enactivism A view of social interaction that rejects an appeal to inner mental states as the primary mediator of intersubjectivity. Rather, social actions are directly coordinated with others' social actions. Regularities in face-to-face interaction are not contingent on knowledge of pre-existing social 'rules' that reside in the minds of interaction partners, but on an outward orientation to the sequence structure of interaction, and participation in one another's sense-making activities. For further reading on enactivism, see De Jaegher and Di Paolo (2007), and for the application of this concept to ASD, see Klin, Jones, Schultz, and Volkmar (2003)

Epistemic resources Express speakers' subjective assessment of the strength of reliability or certainty regarding the truth value of the information in their propositions

Epistemology Relates to the theory of knowledge and what can be known and by what means

First Pair Part (FPP) Is a turn that initiates an action

Forensic patient In the UK, this refers to a patient detained under the Mental Health Act (Department of Health, 2007)

Forensic ward A ward in a secure psychiatric hospital

Foucauldian discourse analysis An approach to discourse analysis that studies historically based ideologies that are assumed to underpin dominant discourses

Frame A structure of expectations which helps people to compartmentalise and recognise regularly encountered types of interaction in the world, for example, institutional discourse, sports, commentary and so on

Genre A constellation of formal features and structures that functions as conventionalised framework for the production and interpretation of discourse, oral as well as written. For further reading, see Briggs and Bauman (1992) and Hanks (1987)

Ideological dilemmas When two or more commonly held beliefs or ideals within a culture appear to contradict each other

Indexicality A pervasive property of language that relates linguistic forms to the contexts in which they are produced. In addition to demonstratives, deictic adverbs and pronouns, many other features of language bear relationship to dimensions of context. For instance, register features relate to a certain professional domain and identity. For further reading on indexicality, see Levinson (1983), and for an in-depth examination of the relationship of this concept to interaction in ASD, see Ochs, Kremer-Sadlik, Sirota, and Solomon (2004)

Interactional sociolinguistics An approach to the study of discourse which analyses power within linguistic practices

Interpretative Phenomenological Analysis Is a method of analysing data where the researcher tries to go beyond what their participant's say and understand their experiences

Intersubjectivity Coordinating or adapting one's subjectivity with other's subjectivity within interaction. A capacity that is embodied prior to becoming reflexive, i.e. a theory of mind (Trevarthen, 1979). For further reading, see Duranti (2010)

Inter-turn pause or gap Is a pause that occurs between syntactic units at a possible transition relevance place

Intra-turn pause Is a pause that occurs within a speaker's turn but not at a possible transition relevance place

Linguistic repertories Ways of talking about a topic that are used by a particular culture or group of people and might include particular phrases, keywords or metaphors that are repeatedly referred to

Minimal response A turn sequential to a question composed of vocal material which indicates little beyond acknowledgement of the prior turn

Neurodevelopmental disorder These are a group of disorders where the brain has developed in a particular way that fundamentally changes the way the brain reacts to the outside world. In turn, this affects particular behaviours and emotions in the person

Nursing assistant A non-qualified practitioner who works with patients under the supervision of qualified staff

Ontology The underpinning theoretical position of a methodological approach. An ontological position is a position on the existence of reality

Orthographic Transcript A transcript that reflects what can be heard in the interviews, but does not include detailed prosodic transcription or other details regarding the delivery of the talk

Paralinguistic Refers to the features which accompany words in a message to convey non-linguistic information, for example, tone, volume, rhythm and so forth

Positive symptoms ofpsychosis An experience that is present that should not be, for example, hearing a voice when there is nobody there

Post-structuralism A label often used to characterise French philosophers and others who generated critiques of structuralism and also argued that for individuals to understand objects, they should study both the object and the systems of knowledge that produce the object—among other beliefs

Recipient design The process in which speakers structure their talk in a way that is sensitive to the particular others involved in the social encounter. For further reading, see Sacks, Schegloff, and Jefferson (1974)

Register A variant of language including both lexical and syntactic choices, associated and identified with a particular context, for example, scientific German, talk directed at pets

Repair A correction of self or other in an interaction to clarify a misunderstanding. This refers to the set of practices whereby interlocutors attend to possible trouble in speaking, hearing or understanding in conversation. For further reading, see Schegloff, Jefferson, and Sacks (1977) and Drew (1997)

Social constructionism This is a theoretical position positing that our understanding of the world is jointly constructed and forms the basis for a shared reality

Social constructivism This is a theoretical position that posits that knowledge is constructed through interaction with others, which emphasises the learning that takes place through interaction

Subject Positions Identities found in discourse, for example, autism as a biological phenomenon that means a person might always be socially awkward, or an autism position that suggests people can high levels of social ability, they just do so differently

Tellability The 'newsworthiness' of a story, as such a fitness criterion for narratives in everyday conversations (Sacks, 1992). For further reading on tellability and narrative in ASD, see Solomon (2004)

Theory of mind This is the appreciation of the views and perspectives of others, the ability to empathise

Therapeutic alliance The collaborative relationship between patient and therapist which enables change

Threshold Concepts Are concepts in learning a discipline that once understood, change a student's way of thinking about a topic

Turn Construction Unit This is a component of a speaker's turn after which the turn may be construed as complete

References

Briggs, C., & Bauman, R. (1992). Genre, intertextuality, and social power. *Journal of Linguistic Anthropology, 2*(2), 131–172.

De Jaegher, H., & Di Paolo, E. (2007). Participatory sense-making. *Phenomenology and Cognitive Science, 6,* 485–507.

Department of Health. (2007). *Mental health act.* London: HMSO.

Drew, P. (1997). 'Open' class repair initiators in response to sequential sources of troubles in conversation. *Journal of Pragmatics, 28,* 69–101.

Duranti, A. (2010). Husserl, intersubjectivity and anthropology. *Anthropological Theory, 10*(1), 1–20.

Edwards, D., & Potter, J. (1992). *Discursive Psychology.* London: Sage.

Hanks, W. (1997). Discourse genres in a theory of practice. *American Ethnologist, 14*(4), 668–692.

Klin, A., Jones, W., Schultz, R., & Volkmar, F. (2003). The enactive mind, or from actions to ognition: Lessons from autism. *Philosophical Transactions of the Royal Society of London B, 358,* 345–360.

Levinson, S. C. (1983). *Pragmatics.* Cambridge: Cambridge University Press.

Ochs, E., Kremer-Sadlik, T., Sirota, K. G., & Solomon, O. (2004). Autism and the social world: An anthropological perspective. *Discourse Studies, 6*(2), 147–182.

Sacks, H. (1992). *Lectures on conversation*. Oxford: Blackwell.

Sacks, H., Schegloff, E. A., & Jefferson, G. (1974). A simplest systematics for the organization of turn-taking for conversation. *Language, 50*(4), 696–735.

Schegloff, E., Jefferson, G., & Sacks, H. (1977). The preference for self-correction in the organisation of repair in conversation. *Language, 53,* 361–382.

Solomon, O. (2004). Narrative introductions: Discourse competence of children with autism spectrum disorders. *Discourse Studies, 6*(2), 253–276.

Trevarthen, C. (1979). Commuincationand cooperation in early infancy: A description of primary intersubjectivity. In M. Buolwa (Ed.), *Before speech: The beginning of interpersonal understanding* (pp. 321–348). Cambridge: Cambridge University Press.

Index

.

Printed by Printforce, the Netherlands

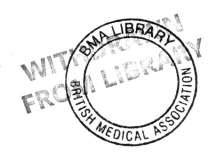